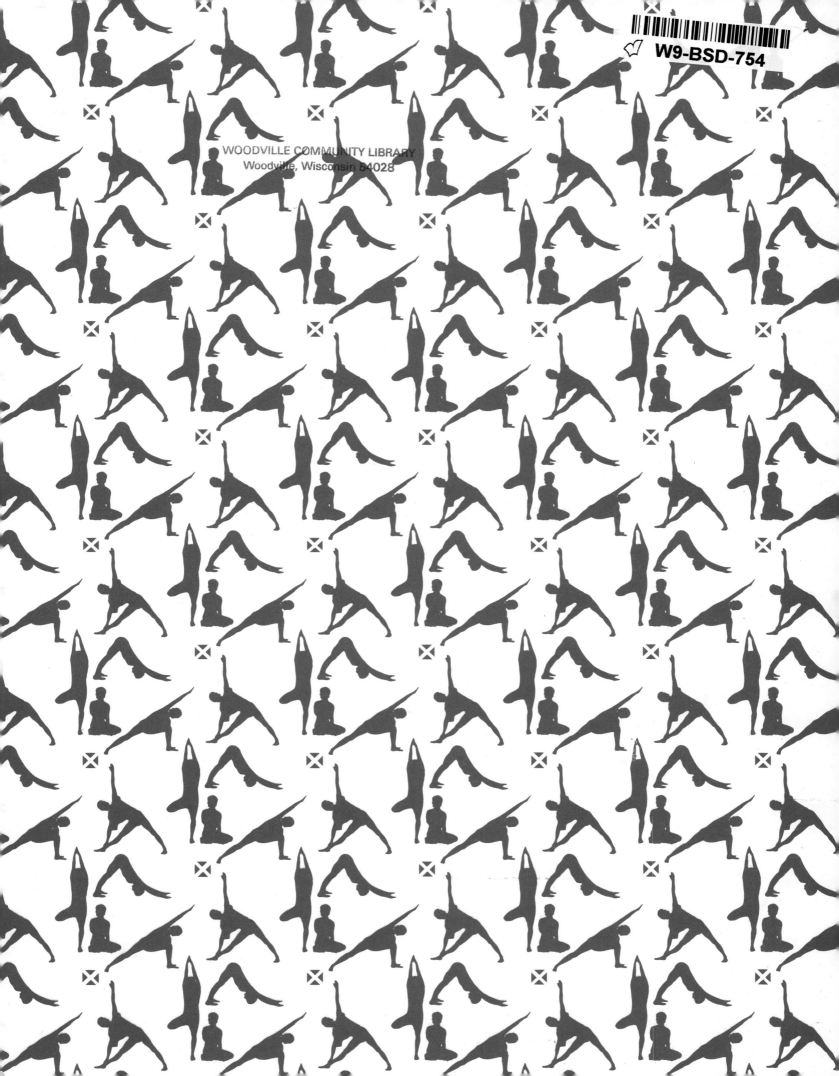

HOW TO USE
YOGA

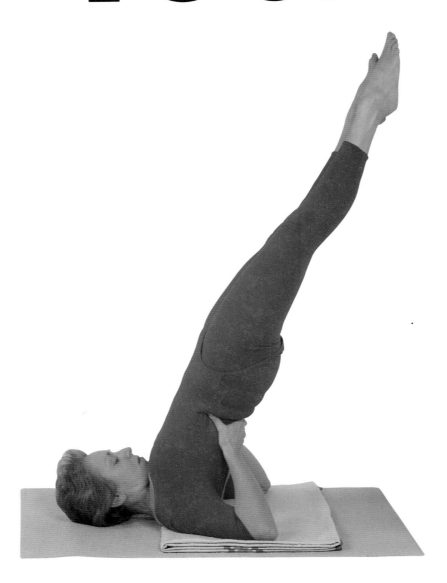

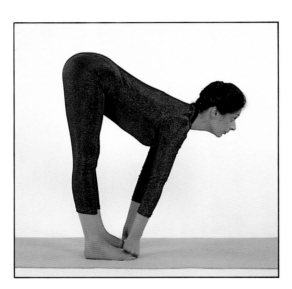
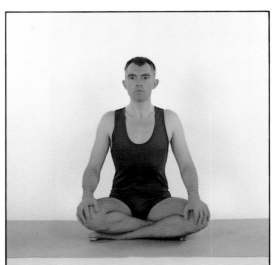
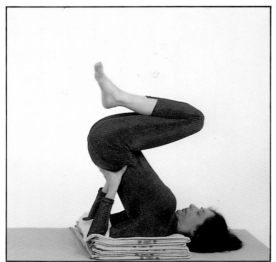
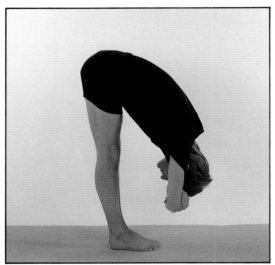

HOW TO USE
YOGA

A step-by-step guide to the Iyengar method of
yoga, for relaxation, health and well-being

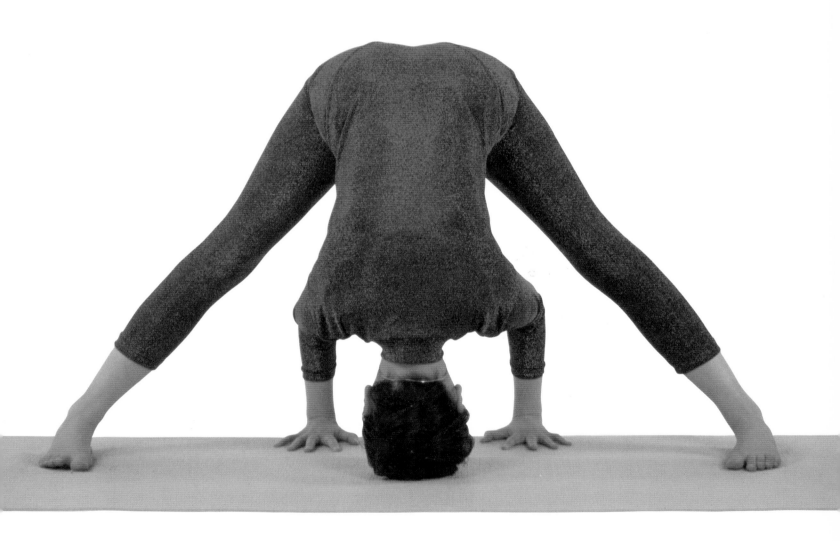

Mira Mehta

SMITHMARK

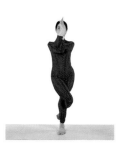

This edition published in 1994 by
SMITHMARK Publishers Inc.
16 East 32nd Street
New York, NY 10016

This book was previously published as part of a larger compendium,
The Encyclopedia of Aromatherapy, Massage and Yoga.

SMITHMARK books are available for bulk purchase
for sales promotion and premium use. For details
write or call the manager of special sales,
SMITHMARK Publishers Inc., 16 East 32nd Street
New York, NY 10016; (212) 532-6600.

Editorial director: Joanna Lorenz
Project editor: Elaine Collins
Photography: Sue Atkinson
Photographic assistant: Kirsty Wilson
Designer: Kit Johnson
Jacket design: Adrian Morris
Artwork: Raymond Turvey, King & King
Typeset by Dorchester Typesetting Group Ltd

Printed and bound in Singapore

ISBN 0-8317-1757-2

ACKNOWLDGEMENTS

The author and publishers would like to thank the following for their
valuable contributions to the book:

Shri B.K.S. Iyengar for the advice on the text, The Iyengar Yoga
Institute for providing advice, expertise and personnel, Juliet Algie,
Paula Clark, Eric Haines, Maria Johnson, Mira Mehta, Glenys
Shepherd, David Tierney and Ormond Uren for appearing in the
photographs, and Gerry List Photography for the pictures appearing
on pages 8 and 9.

CONTENTS

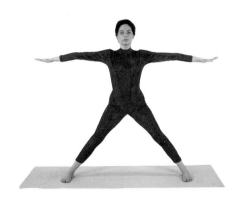

THE IYENGAR BASICS 6

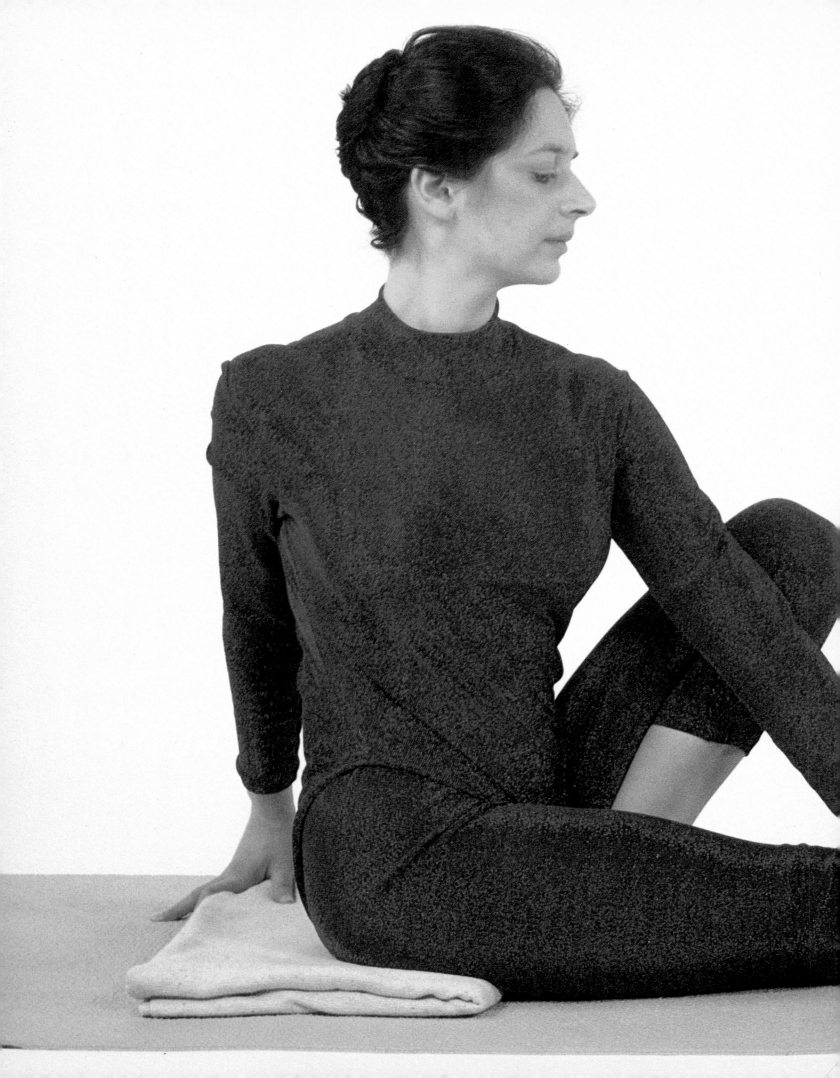

YOGA
THE IYENGAR BASICS

A powerful antidote to the stresses of modern-day life, yoga is a practical philosophy that aims at uniting the body, mind and spirit for health and fulfilment. A fit and supple body can be developed through the practice of postures (asanas). These easy-to-follow exercises, especially chosen for beginners, work on all the bodily systems, toning the muscles, stimulating the circulation and improving overall health. The benefits are not merely physical: as the postures are mastered and techniques introduced for relaxation and breath control, you will find that yoga has the power to calm the mind, increase your concentration and give the ability to cope with tension. It is a complete system for personal development, promoting total physical and spiritual well-being.

The authors wish to acknowledge their indebtedness to Yogacharya Sri B.K.S. Iyengar for his help and support in the preparation of this work.

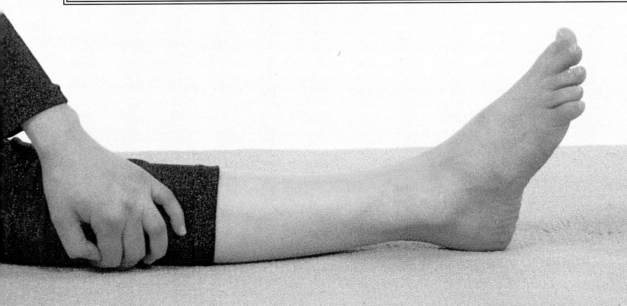

THE GIFT OF YOGA

Yoga is one of India's wonderful gifts to mankind. One of its valuable qualities is that it builds up a store of physical health through the practice of a system of exercises called asanas which keep the body cleansed and fit. Yoga believes that exercise is essential for speedy removal of toxins and for keeping blood circulation and all internal processes functioning smoothly.

Having dealt with the physical side of life, yoga turns to the mental. Here different breathing exercises or techniques quieten the mind and brain, offering inner peace and an ability to face upheavals and deal with problems.

Uniting both these aspects is the philosophy of yoga which has stood the test of time, bidding humanity to review its thinking and its conduct, and to turn away from violence, dishonesty and greed – a review of life much needed in the present day.

Yoga therefore has a role both in everyday practical life, and in the more thoughtful, idealistic scheme of things. Its value needs to be experienced and savoured.

YOGA – A BRIEF OVERVIEW

Yoga has been practised in India for over two millenia. Stories and legends from ancient times all testify to the existence of yoga, and to the practitioners and divinities associated with it.

Indian literature is a storehouse of knowledge about yoga covering every conceivable level. Roughly in chronological order are the *Vedas* (books of scriptural knowledge), the *Upanisads* (philosophical speculations), and their commentaries; then the *Puranas* (ancient cosmologies), and the two epics, the *Ramayana* and the *Mahabharata*. The *Mahabharata* contains within itself that masterpiece of Indian scripture, the *Bhagavad Gita*. Toward the end of the Vedic period comes the aphoristic literature, with the "Yoga Aphorisms" of Patanjali of especial interest to yoga students. There are, besides, whole bodies of works both ancient (pre-Christian) and more modern dealing with various aspects of yoga and yoga philosophy, testifying to the continued relevance of yoga as a discipline.

Yoga is considered to be a philosophy, a science and an art. It has eight clearly defined aspects and, in its purest form, is a complete system capable of answering all human needs. However, it has always been, and still is, used as a basis for other activities and disciplines. Today, for example, physiotherapy and exercise classes often adapt movements from yoga postures.

Different schools of yoga through the ages have

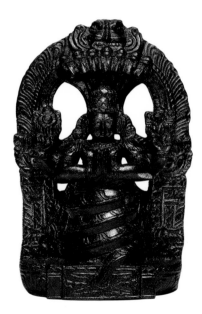

Patanjali is the legendary founder of yoga. According to tradition he brought to humanity serenity of spirit through the philosophy of yoga, clarity of speech by his work on grammar, and health of body by his work on medicine.

Indian iconography gives him a half human, half serpent form, as depicted in this modern sculpture.

stressed different aspects, but all branches have a common ideological basis, of seeking the betterment of individual yoga practitioners, and, in a broader context, of humanity.

The word yoga comes from the Sanskrit root *"yuj"* meaning to join or yoke, implying the integration (or joining) of every aspect of a human being from the innermost to the external. Another frequently used definition of yoga is that of union of the individual spirit with the universal, since that is its highest aim.

As a philosophy, yoga is unusual in that it insists that the practice of postures – apparently physical exercises – and breathing techniques is essential in order to lead a worthy and satisfying life. A whole doctrine attaches to the postural and breathing aspects of yoga. The parallel classical Western concept of *"mens sana in corpore sano"* – a healthy body in a healthy mind – has always been recognized and is finding increasing emphasis today.

PATANJALI AND THE YOGA SUTRAS

The first semi-historical, semi-mythological figure in yoga is that of the sage Patanjali who lived some time in the pre-Christian era – one estimate suggests about 220 BC. He is traditionally said to be the author of works on medicine, grammar and yoga. Together these cover the fields of the body, the intellect and the spirit. His treatise on yoga is called the "Yoga Sutras" or "Yoga Aphorisms" and it is still considered authoritative today.

The *Yoga Sutras* summarizes all the various aspects of yoga and systematizes them. According to Patanjali, yoga consists of eight limbs, which are all equally important and are related as parts of a whole. They are as follows:

1. Five universal commandments (*yama*) aimed at creating a "better" world: not harming anyone or anything; truthfulness; non-stealing; leading a godly, chaste life; and being non-grasping.

2. Five personal disciplines (*niyama*): cleanliness; contentedness; self-discipline; self-study and study of the scriptures; and dedication to God.

3. Practice of postures (*asana*): devoted and conscientious practice of the various types of posture.

4. Practice of breath control (*pranayama*): practising breathing techniques with care and discrimination.

5. Detachment from worldly activities (*pratyahara*): developing a non-attached attitude of body and mind.

6. Concentration (*dharana*): Being able to hold on to a subject mentally.

7. Meditation (*dhyana*): developing a quiet, meditative state.

8. Trance or a state of bliss (*samadhi*): reaching a state of absorption in a subject or in the Divine.

THE INFLUENCE OF B.K.S. IYENGAR

 he work of B.K.S. Iyengar confirms him as a modern pioneer of yoga. He has explained and exemplified all the traditional aspects of the subject as laid down by Patanjali. He has rediscovered and systematized a whole range of postures and breathing techniques, making them accessible to yoga practitioners of all levels, throughout the world.

Most importantly, B.K.S. Iyengar has worked extensively on the therapeutic effects of yoga. His authority is acknowledged throughout the world by all schools of yoga and his books *Light on Yoga* and *Light on Pranayama* are modern classics. He has received numerous titles and awards for his services to yoga from the Government of India and from various educational organizations.

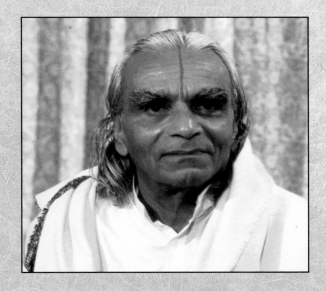

The postures and breath control techniques given in this book are based on B.K.S. Iyengar's work.

TOWARD PHYSICAL WELLBEING

Yoga is an ineffable art which, though backed by a very logical philosophy, does not reveal itself by theorization. Only by practice does one experience the effects of the various asanas and pranayamas on the body, mind and spirit.

Why the body becomes supple and efficient through yoga can easily be understood. Why and how yoga affects the mind is not so immediately apparent. But why it should affect the spirit – will-power, feeling of well-being, energy – seems to defy all logic.

On reading this you may think, "This is all very interesting, but it is not for me". However, if you practise some of the postures in the way they have been described, you are likely to be agreeably surprised. Although you may find that the postures are more difficult than they look, and not all your joints may be working as well as you expected, do not give up. The postures will soon begin to help you with any physical weaknesses you may have. They will also stretch your mind and enhance your concentration.

SCOPE OF THE COURSE

The aim of this course is to provide a basic introduction to the theory and practice of yoga. The major part, *Toward Physical Wellbeing*, deals with 41 postures and variants – the Asanas – which may be attempted by beginners of all ages. Principal techniques are given with clear illustrations and stages so that the postures may be easily followed by everyone.

A ten-week course is included to guide your practice systematically and progressively. Daily practice is suggested, but if you cannot do this the course will take longer. A few necessary precautions are given to make sure your practice will be safe. Some general practice points are also given.

In addition, there is a section giving postures which are helpful for some common problems – headaches, stiffness and pain in the neck and shoulders, backache and stiffness of the hips. There is also a programme of postures suitable to be done during menstruation.

In *Toward Mental Peace*, guidance is given in some simple relaxation and breathing techniques to show how these calm the mind.

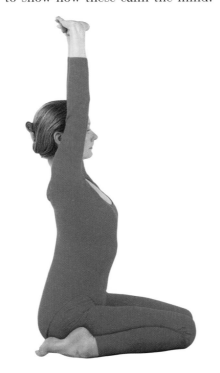

HOME PRACTICE

There are several ways of planning practice at home. These depend on a number of factors such as time available, family and other duties, and individual requirements.

Time

There are no set rules about when to practise, or how long. Clearly the more yoga is done, the greater the benefit.

Some people prefer to practise in the morning, others in the evening. It is also possible to break up practice sessions so that they slot in to shorter periods whenever is convenient during the day – even if only for 10 minutes at a time.

Family and other Duties

Practice may be modified according to circumstances. At times it may need to be geared to fulfilling family and other obligations effectively. In this case it is important to plan the time and programme for practice carefully so as to derive maximum benefit. For example, if you have only 10 or 20 minutes to spare and are being faced with a heavy workload or stressful situation, supported Sarvangasana (nos. 37 and 38) and Setu Bandha Sarvangasana (no. 39) or Viparita Karani (no. 40) may be the most appropriate.

Level

The practice of postures and pranayama will vary according to the level and experience of the student. The basic poses should be practised on a regular basis and should never be forgotten. One method is to vary the type of postures done each day, for instance, standing poses one day and sitting poses the next. Always include inverted poses. Beginners should concentrate more on standing poses.

Individual Needs

In home practice you have to be sensitive to your own needs and to be aware which postures are helpful in different circumstances. For example, standing poses are invigorating, whereas forward bends are calming.

This is one approach to practice. The other is to discipline yourself to do a particular programme irrespective of personal inclination. The first approach makes you sensitive and the second develops will-power. Both need to be learnt.

Where there is a health problem for which a certain group of postures are prescribed, then this particular programme should be adhered to.

Structure

Yoga practice should have a structure. A basic guide is to start with simple poses or those which allow the body to stretch; then to continue with the main group or groups of poses selected for that day, and to end with relaxing poses that allow the work done to be assimilated by the body.

Self-discipline

Practising at home requires and develops self-discipline and an independent understanding of the postures. It is a good idea to begin by remembering some of the postures and instructions given. The building up of correct habits will give a firm foundation in yoga, leading to confidence in practice and greater knowledge.

Repetition of Postures

It is usual to repeat some of the postures when practising, such as standing poses, sitting poses and twists, so long as this does not cause fatigue. However, do not repeat the inverted postures and recuperative positions.

Timings in the Postures

Guidance is given in the Asana section for the timing of each posture. In the beginning do not stay long in the postures, until they become familiar and you gain stamina. Do not strain to hold a posture. Gradually increase the time spent in each so that the postures – as well as your health – improve.

Breathing in the Postures

Do upward movements with an inhalation, downward movements with an exhalation. That is, start a movement at the beginning of an inhalation or exhalation, and conclude it at the end of the same breath if possible. Do not hold the breath in the postures.

Menstruation

Women should not do inverted poses during menstruation as these interfere with the natural outflow of blood. There is a whole range of postures which are suitable at this time – see Asanas for Menstruation.

=======CAUTION=======

This course is not intended for those suffering from the following conditions:
- cancer or benign tumours
- detached retina
- diabetes
- epilepsy including petit mal
- heart disease
- high blood pressure
- HIV
- Meniere's disease
- Multiple Sclerosis (MS)
- Myalgic Encephalomyelitis (ME)
- physical handicaps
- pregnancy
- recent post-operative conditions

In such cases, please seek the advice of an experienced teacher.

THE ASANAS

There are many different types of yoga postures – Indian texts sometimes mention 840,000! – but in practice only about 20 or 30 principal ones were in regular use until recently. However, through the work of B.K.S. Iyengar, over 200 postures are now being practised by yoga students all over the world. The system of postures has come to be accepted as a subject in its own right, since great attention is paid to the precision and correct execution of the movements.

The postures (asanas) are all anatomically and physiologically sound. They are a guide to the variety of movement attainable by the human body. In the Iyengar method they have been categorized according to level of difficulty, to be practised by those from beginner level to advanced stages.

The postures are grouped according to the positioning of the body – standing, sitting, twisting, prone, supine, inverted and balancing. They incorporate slow and quick motion and teach concentration, dynamism and stillness. They have important therapeutic effects, since the entire organic structure is invigorated and toned by practice of the postures. Muscle tone is automatically improved. The yoga student will benefit from increasing health, stamina and agility.

At the psychological level, the postures have their own intrinsic value since they are challenging and interesting to do. They also have a direct balancing effect on certain psychological disorders – thus, they can "liven up" a lethargic and depressed person, or calm a frenetic, distressed person.

BEFORE YOU BEGIN

There are some basic guidelines which should be followed before beginning yoga practice:

● Wait for 4–5 hours after a heavy meal or 2–3 hours after a light snack.

● Empty the bladder and move the bowels before you start. Supported Sarvangasana (no. 38) and Ardha Halasana (no. 36) will help.

● Practise in loose-fitting clothing and bare feet.

● Work on a non-slip mat or floor. Especially in the winter, the floor should not be too cold.

● Fold blankets neatly when preparing to use them, as any creases will disturb your practice.

● Remove hard contact lenses.

● Seek advice if you experience difficulties in practice. Your difficulty may be a common one, and there is likely to be a solution. In the meantime, avoid straining.

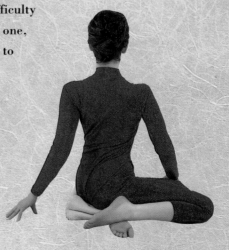

STANDING POSES

1 · TADASANA
MOUNTAIN POSE

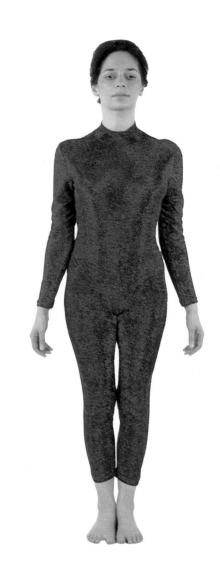

*This is the first posture to be learnt. It is the basic standing pose,
with which they start and finish.*

*Although Tadasana is practised from the beginning, it is difficult to master
as it involves bringing the energies of the body and mind into equilibrium in
a static pose. This can only be done when postural defects have been
corrected by working on a variety of asanas. For this reason, beginners
should become familiar with the postures gradually.*

Stand with the feet together, and big toes, heels and ankle bones touching. Keep the knees straight and pull up the thigh muscles. Stretch the legs up, extend the spine and lift the front of the body. Take the shoulders back, shoulder blades in and allow the arms to hang loosely at the sides of the trunk. Relax the hands and keep the palms facing the hips. Extend the neck up and relax the face. Look straight ahead. Concentrate on centering the body: balance the weight evenly on both feet; create awareness in the soles of the feet and stretch them equally. Be conscious of extending the right and left sides of the body evenly. Keep the chest open.

Stay in the posture for 30–60 seconds when practising Tadasana on its own; less when doing it as a stage of other poses.

NOTES ON THE POSTURES

Read the following notes regarding individual groups of postures before beginning practice.

Standing poses
● Do not jump into the postures if you have a bad back or injured knees.
● Do not strain the knees when straightening them.
● Do not hold the breath.
● Do not strain the throat or the abdomen.

Sitting poses
● Sit on one or two folded blankets in order not to strain the lower back. Reduce the height when you are more flexible.
● Do not use force to straighten the legs but extend them carefully.

Twists
● Sit on folded blankets to raise the base of the spine. You will then be able to turn the whole trunk.
● Do not tense the abdomen.

Inverted poses
● Avoid these postures during menstruation. Postures to be done at this time are given in the section – "Asanas for Menstruation".
● These poses should feel comfortable. If you experience pressure in any part of the head or neck, your blankets may need adjusting, or you may have gone up awkwardly.
● Seek advice if you have or have had any head or neck injuries, or any medical condition affecting the eyes, ears or brain.

2 · VRKSASANA
TREE POSE

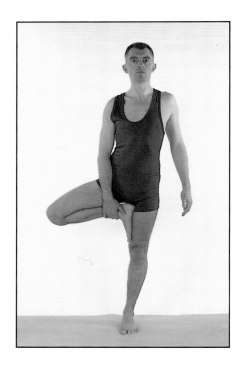

1 *Stand in Tadasana (no. 1). Without disturbing the left leg, bend the right leg to the side. Catch the ankle and place the foot at the top of the inner left thigh. Take it as high as possible. Press the right knee back, in line with the right hip.*

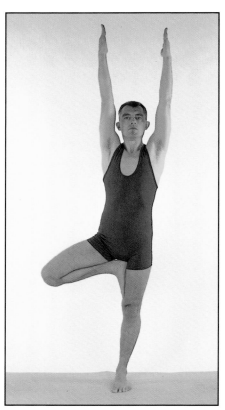

2 *Inhale and take the arms over the head with the palms facing each other. Straighten the elbows and stretch the arms and trunk up. Stand firmly on the left foot so that you do not overbalance. Stretch the leg up.*

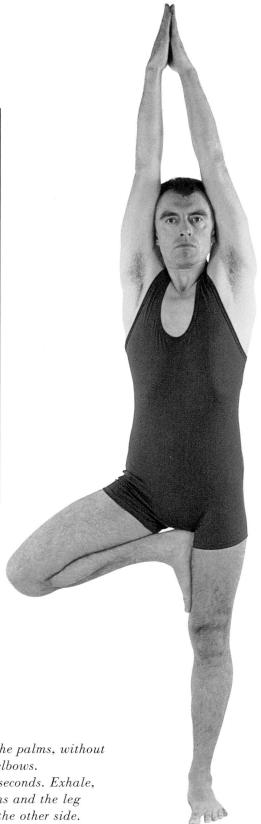

3 *Right: Join the palms, without bending the elbows.*
Stay for 20–30 seconds. Exhale, then bring the arms and the leg down. Repeat on the other side.

3 · UTTHITA TRIKONASANA
— EXTENDED TRIANGLE POSE —

Trikonasana is one of the most important standing poses. Learn the various points gradually, incorporate them into your practice and build on them.

● *If you have a bad back or injured knees, do not jump into standing poses.*

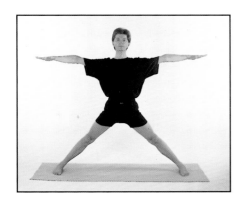

1 Stand in Tadasana (no. 1). With a deep inhalation, jump the feet about 3½–4 ft (105–120 cm) apart, at the same time raising the arms to shoulder level, palms face down. Line up the feet to be level and facing forward.

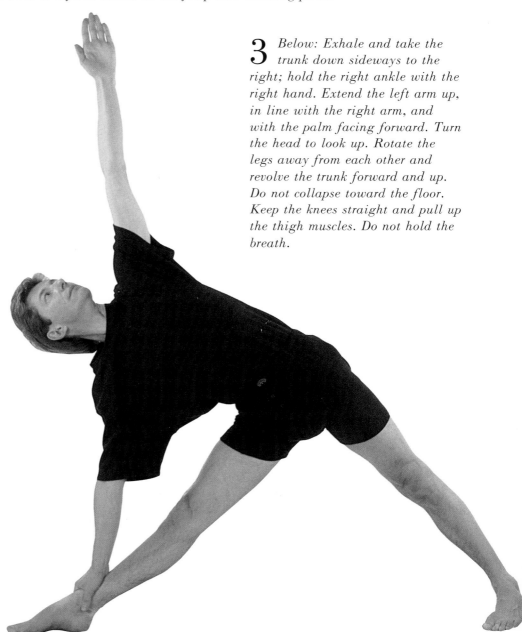

3 *Below: Exhale and take the trunk down sideways to the right; hold the right ankle with the right hand. Extend the left arm up, in line with the right arm, and with the palm facing forward. Turn the head to look up. Rotate the legs away from each other and revolve the trunk forward and up. Do not collapse toward the floor. Keep the knees straight and pull up the thigh muscles. Do not hold the breath.*

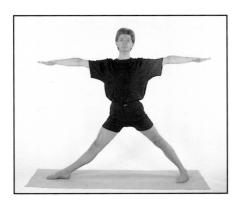

2 Turn the left foot about 15° in and the right foot about 90° out. Line up the right heel to be exactly opposite the left instep. As you turn the left foot in, rotate the left leg outwards. As you turn the right foot out, rotate the whole leg in the same direction (that is, to the right). Keep the knees tight and lift the trunk.

Stay for 20–30 seconds. Inhale and come up to 2. Turn the feet to the centre. Rest the arms for a moment so that you do not feel fatigue (you may place them on the hips). Line up the feet again. Repeat on the other side. Come up, then exhale, jump the feet together and bring the arms down.

4 · UTTHITA PARSVAKONASANA
EXTENDED LATERAL ANGLE POSE

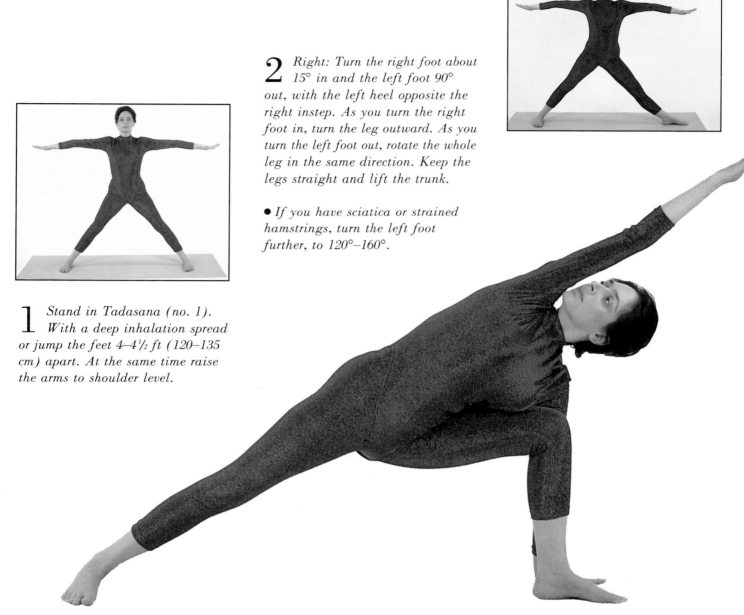

2 *Right: Turn the right foot about 15° in and the left foot 90° out, with the left heel opposite the right instep. As you turn the right foot in, turn the leg outward. As you turn the left foot out, rotate the whole leg in the same direction. Keep the legs straight and lift the trunk.*

● *If you have sciatica or strained hamstrings, turn the left foot further, to 120°–160°.*

1 *Stand in Tadasana (no. 1). With a deep inhalation spread or jump the feet 4–4½ ft (120–135 cm) apart. At the same time raise the arms to shoulder level.*

3 *Keep the right leg firm and bend the left leg to 90°, with the shin perpendicular and the thigh parallel to the ground. Exhale and take the trunk sideways down to the left. Bend from the hips, not the waist. Place the left palm or fingertips on the floor by the outer edge of the left foot.*

Turn the right arm and stretch it over the head, palm face down. Turn the head and look up. Keeping the right leg and both arms straight, revolve the whole trunk upward. Stretch the right side of the body toward the fingertips. Relax the face and breathe normally.
Stay for 20–30 seconds. Inhale

and come up. Turn the feet to the centre and rest the arms on the hips. Repeat on the other side. Come up to step 2, then exhale, and jump back to Tadasana.

● *If breathing becomes strained, come up and rest, or face the ground till the breath returns to normal.*

5 · VIRABHADRASANA I
WARRIOR POSE I

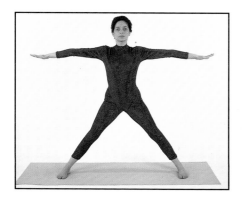

1 Stand in Tadasana (no. 1). With a deep inhalation, spread or jump the feet 4–4½ ft (120–135 cm) apart, raising the arms to shoulder level.

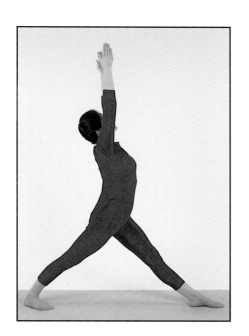

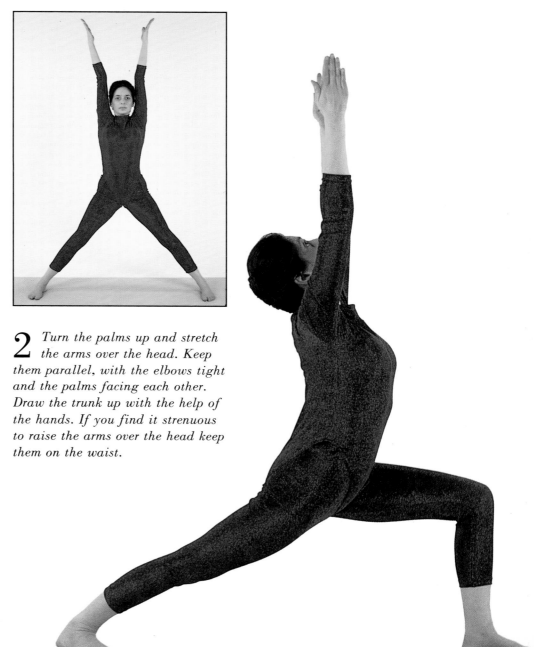

2 Turn the palms up and stretch the arms over the head. Keep them parallel, with the elbows tight and the palms facing each other. Draw the trunk up with the help of the hands. If you find it strenuous to raise the arms over the head keep them on the waist.

3 Turn the right leg and foot 45° in, and the left foot 90° out. At the same time turn the hips and trunk to the left. Make the left and right sides of the body parallel by bringing the right hip forward and taking the left hip slightly further back.

4 Exhale and bend the left leg to a right angle. Stretch the whole body up. Move the shoulder blades in and open the chest. Take the head back and look up. Do not strain the neck and throat. Keep the back leg firm and maintain the turn of the hips and trunk to the left. Stretch up to the maximum.

Stay for 20–30 seconds. Inhale and come up. Turn to the centre. Rest the arms and line up the feet. Repeat on the other side. Come up, then exhale and jump into Tadasana.

6. VIRABHADRASANA II
WARRIOR POSE II

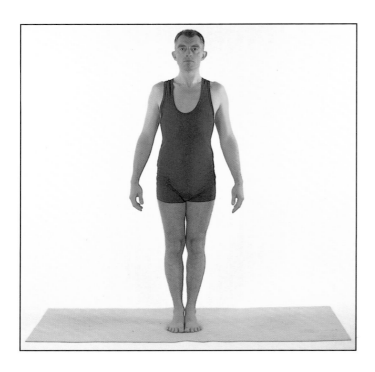

1   *Stand in Tadasana (no. 1).*

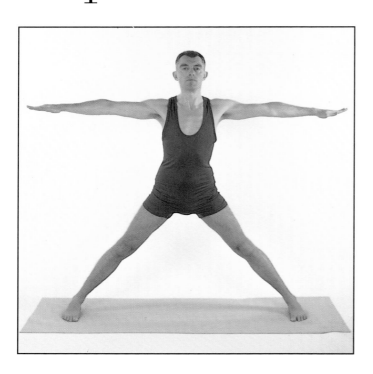

2   *With a deep inhalation spread or jump the feet 4–4½ ft (120–135 cm) apart, raising the arms to shoulder level.*

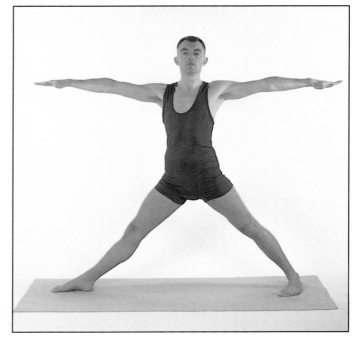

3   *Turn the left foot about 15° in and the right foot 90° out. Line up the feet, with the right heel opposite the left instep. While turning the left foot in, rotate the left leg outward. While turning the right foot out, rotate the whole leg together with the foot. Keep both knees tight. Lift up the trunk from the hips.*

● *If you have sciatica, turn the right foot 120°–160°.*

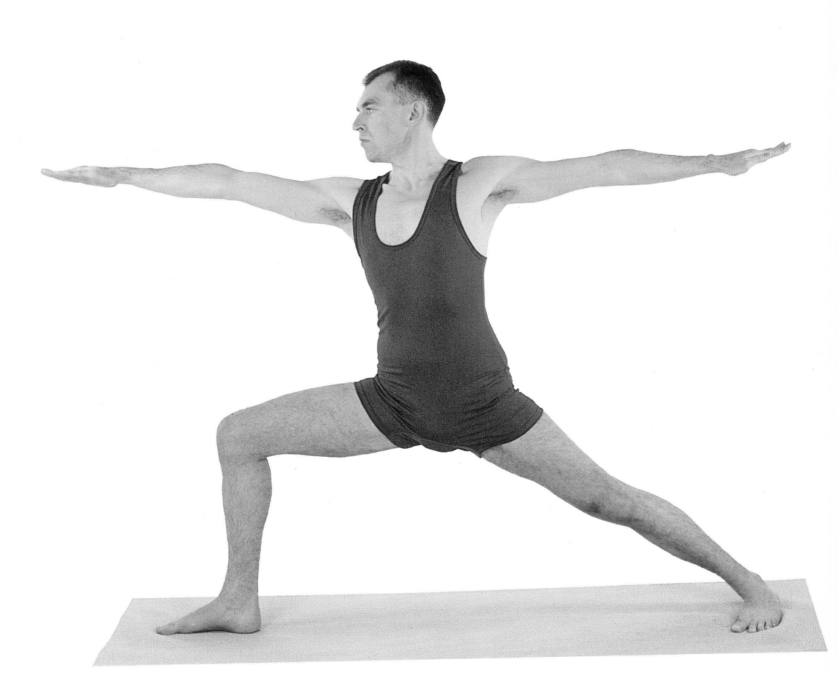

4 *With an exhalation, bend the right leg to a right angle, keeping the left leg straight. Extend the trunk vertically up and stretch the arms horizontally to the sides, palms face down. Turn the head to the right. Pull the left arm slightly to the left so that the trunk does not lean to the right. Lift the chest. Relax the face and breathe normally.*

Stay for 20–30 seconds. Inhale and come up. Turn the feet to the centre and line them up. Rest the arms if necessary.

Repeat on the other side. Come up, then exhale and jump into Tadasana.

7. PARSVOTTANASANA
EXTREME SIDEWAYS STRETCH

FULL POSE

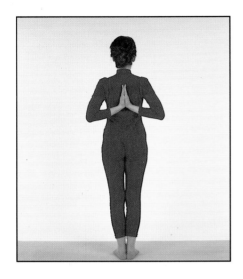

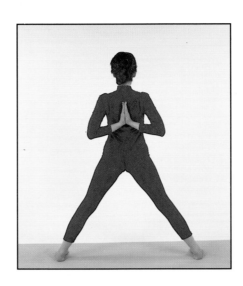

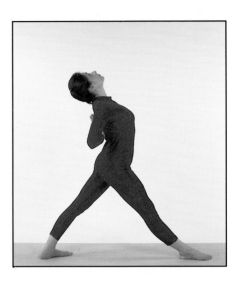

1 Stand in Tadasana (no. 1). Join the palms behind the back in Namaste (for method, see box on facing page).

2 With a deep inhalation, jump the feet 3½– 4 ft (105–120 cm) apart. Line up the toes to make them level.

3 Turn the left leg and foot about 45° in, and the right foot 90° out. Turn the hips and trunk to the right. Stretch the trunk up and take the head back. Do not strain the throat.

4 Right: Exhale and bend down over the right leg. Keep both legs straight and make the hips level. Stretch down as far as you can, then relax the head.

   Stay for 20–30 seconds. Inhale and come up. Turn to the front, without releasing the hands. Line up the feet, then repeat on the other side.

   Come up, turn to the front, then exhale and jump into Tadasana. Finally, bring the hands down.

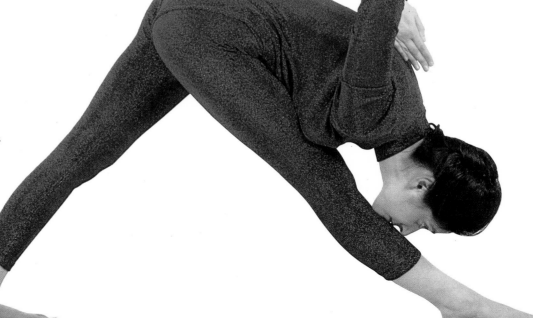

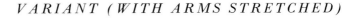

VARIANT (SIMPLE)

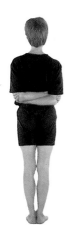

In step 1 (Tadasana), instead of joining the palms behind the back in Namaste, catch the elbows.

VARIANT (WITH ARMS STRETCHED)

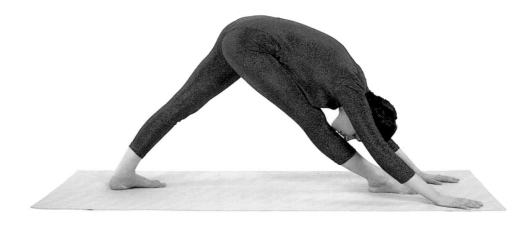

Instead of taking the arms back, stretch them up over the head and then take the trunk and arms down over the leg. Rest the hands on the floor, on either side of the front foot. In this position it is easier to balance and to keep the extension of the trunk.

NAMASTE
HANDS IN PRAYER POSITION

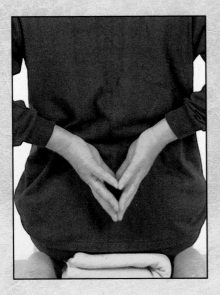

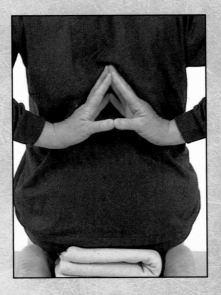

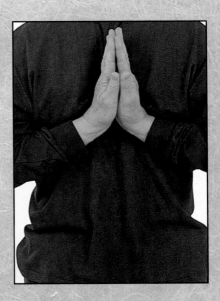

1 *Join the palms behind the back, with the fingers pointing down.*

2 *Turn the hands toward the spine.*

3 *Turn the hands up and raise them between the shoulder blades. Take the shoulders and elbows back and press the palms together.*

8 · PRASARITA PADOTTANASANA
FORWARD STRETCH WITH LEGS WIDE APART

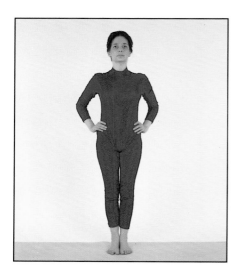

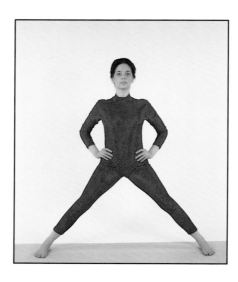

3 *Below: Bend down and place the hands on the floor, shoulder width apart, with the arms slanting back a little. Straighten the arms. Keep the legs firm. Make the back concave and extend the front of the body forward. Look up.*

Bend the elbows back, lower the trunk and place the crown of the head on the floor. If possible take the hands further back, in line with the feet. Lift the hips and the shoulders. Relax and breathe evenly.

Stay for 20–30 seconds. Inhale, raise the head and make the spine concave. Then place the hands on the hips and come up. Bring the feet in a little and jump them together.

1 *Stand in Tadasana (no. 1), with the hands on the hips.*

2 *With a deep inhalation, jump the feet 4½–5 ft (135–150 cm) apart. Line them up. Turn them to face forward or slightly in so that you do not slip. Straighten the legs and pull up the thigh muscles.*

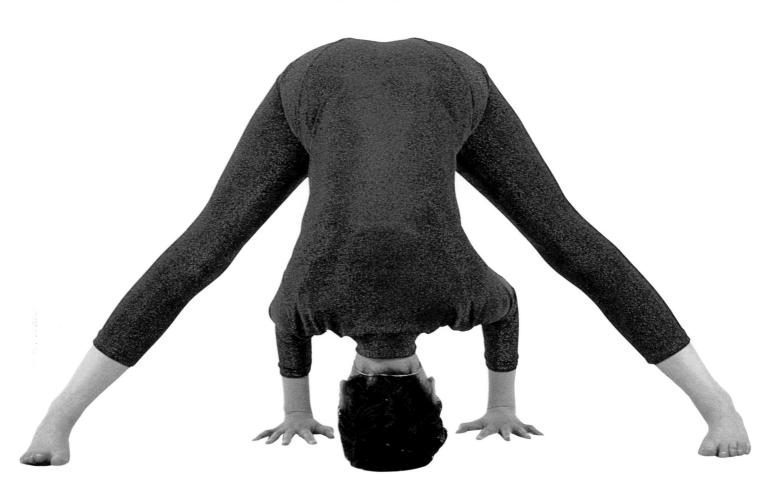

9 · UTTANASANA
FORWARD EXTENSION

Stand in Tadasana (no. 1) with the feet about 1 ft (30 cm) apart. Catch the elbows and take the arms over the head. Draw the waist slightly back. Stretch the legs up strongly.

Exhale and bend down. Bring the hips and chest as close to the legs as possible and if you can, go on extending until the head reaches beyond the knees. Pull on the elbows to bring the trunk further down. Bring the hips further forward to make the legs vertical. Keep the knees straight and the leg muscles pulled up. Relax the head and breathe evenly.

Stay for 20–30 seconds. Inhale, come up and bring the legs together.

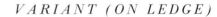

NOTE

If you feel dizzy, or have a bad back, do Uttanasana with the hands on a ledge instead.

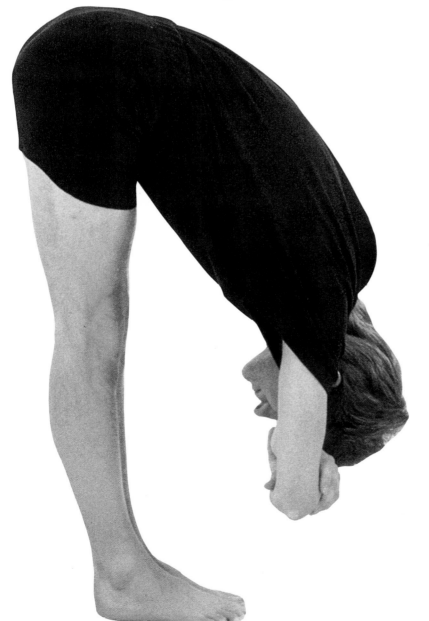

VARIANT (ON LEDGE)

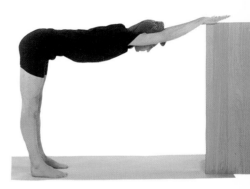

Stand facing a ledge 4–5 ft (120–150 cm) away. Take the feet about 1 ft (30 cm) apart. Bend forward and place the hands on the ledge. Adjust your distance by stepping closer or further away as necessary to enable the legs to be vertical and the trunk and arms to be extended.

Straighten the legs, tighten the kneecaps and pull up the thigh muscles. Extend the arms and the trunk forward. Take the hips further down and make the upper back concave.

Stay for 20–30 seconds.

10 · PADANGUSTHASANA
FINGER-TO-FOOT POSE

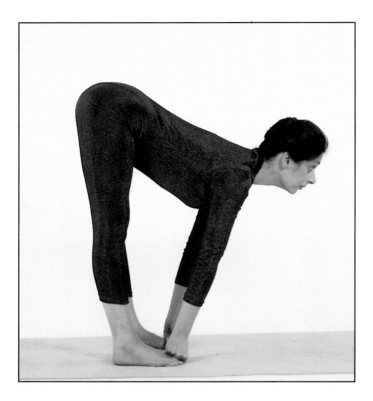

1 Stand with the feet about 1 ft (30 cm) apart. Bend down and make a ring round the big toes with the thumb, index and middle fingers. Straighten the knees and stretch the legs vertically up. Straighten the arms, extend the trunk forward and make the back concave. Look up.

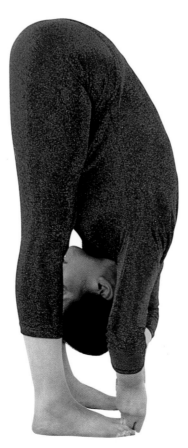

2 Right: Exhale, bend the elbows outward, pull the trunk down and bring the head towards the shins.
   Stay for 20–30 seconds. Inhale and come up, then join the feet and stand erect.

11 · GARUDASANA
EAGLE POSE

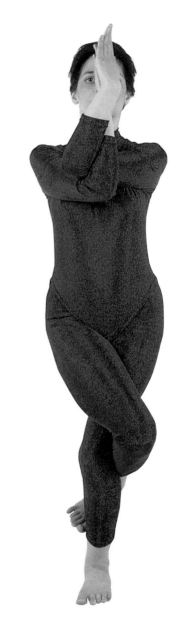

Stand in Tadasana (no. 1). Bend the left leg a little. Bend the right leg and cross the thigh over the left. Swing the right foot back and hook it round the left calf.
   Bend the elbows and raise them to shoulder level, with the thumbs pointing to the face. Cross the left elbow over the right, then hook the right wrist and palm over the left.
   Stay for 20–30 seconds, then repeat on the other side.

12 · UTKATASANA
─── FIERCE POSE ───

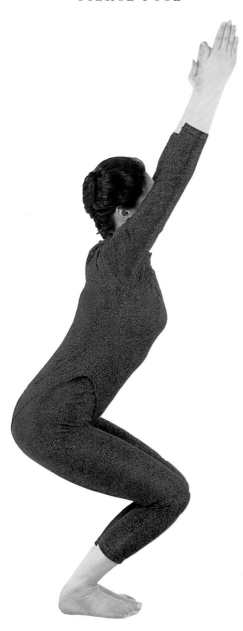

Stand in Tadasana (no. 1). Inhale
and stretch the arms over the head,
with the palms facing each other.
Straighten the elbows and stretch
the palms and fingers. Use the
hands to pull the trunk up strongly.
Bend the knees and take the hips
back as if preparing to sit. Bend
more in the ankle joints and press
the heels down. If you can keep the
elbows straight, join the palms.

Stay for 20–30 seconds, then
come up.

13 · UTTHITA HASTA PADANGUSTHASANA
─── LEG RAISING ───

FORWARD

Stand in Tadasana (no. 1),
facing a ledge 2–3 ft (60–90
cm) away. Bend the right leg
and place the back of the heel
(not the Achilles tendon) on the
ledge, directly in front of you.
Keep the knee and big toe facing
the ceiling. Stretch the left leg
and keep the foot facing
forward. Straighten both the
knees. Extend the right leg and
heel away from you. Stretch the
left leg and the trunk vertically
up. Rest the hands at the sides
of the trunk, on the hips or
stretch them up.

Stay for 20–30 seconds, then
come down and repeat on the
other side.

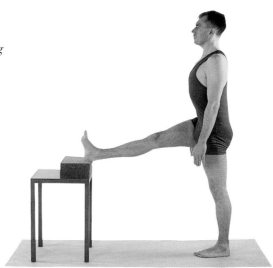

SIDEWAYS

Stand in Tadasana (no. 1), 2–3
ft (60–90 cm) away from a
ledge and sideways to it. Bend
the right leg outward and place
the heel on the ledge, in line
with the outer hip. Keep the left
leg perpendicular and the foot
facing forward. Tighten the
kneecaps and the thigh muscles.
Stretch the right leg out to the
side and stretch the trunk and
the left leg upward. Place the
hands on the hips or stretch them
above the head.

Stay for 20–30 seconds, then
take the foot down and repeat on
the other side.

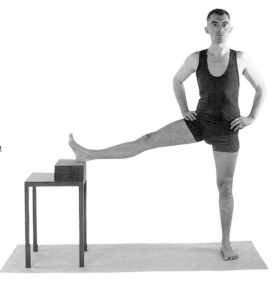

SITTING POSES

14 · SUKHASANA

— *EASY POSE* —

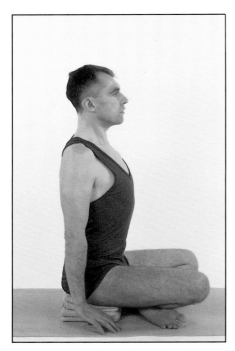

1 *Sit on one or two folded blankets in simple cross-legs. Cross the shins, not only the ankles. Place the hands beside the hips, press the fingertips into the ground and extend the trunk up. Open the chest and take the shoulders back.*

2 *Maintain the trunk erect and bring the hands on to the knees.*
   Stay for 30–60 seconds, then change the cross-legs and repeat.

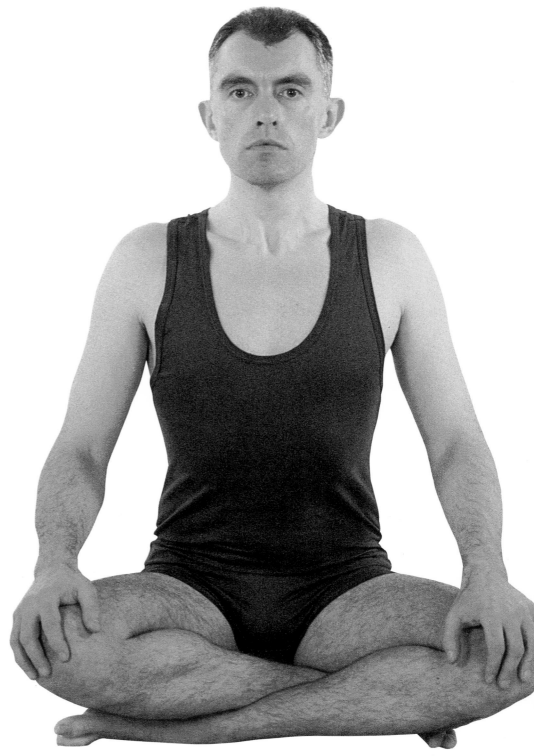

15 · VIRASANA
HERO POSE

The knees should be comfortable in this posture. If you have weak or injured knees, fold a piece of cloth and place it behind the knee joint to create space; or sit on a bolster and learn to flex the knees. For other problems, seek advice.

Kneel with the knees together and the feet apart beside the hips. Sit between the legs, on a height of folded blankets if necessary.

Stretch the trunk up. Take the shoulders back and broaden them. Roll the inner thighs outward to take the outer thighs down and bring the shins closer to the thighs. Rest the hands on the legs.

Stay for 1–2 minutes, then come out of the posture and straighten the legs.

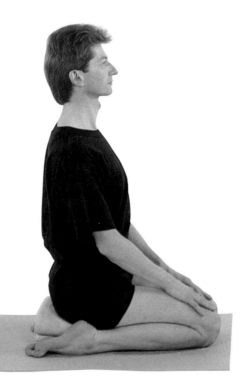

16 · VIRASANA FORWARD BEND
HERO POSE WITH FORWARD BEND

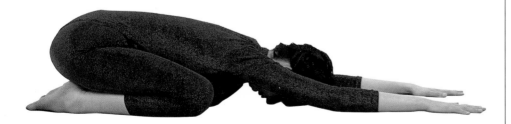

Sit between the legs or on the heels. If the buttocks do not rest easily on the heels, place a folded blanket or bolster on the heels. Spread the knees slightly apart and bend down. Stretch the chest and the arms forward and keep the sides of the body touching the inner thighs; do not spread the legs too wide apart.

17 · PARVATASANA
MOUNTAIN POSE

This posture can be done in several sitting positions, such as Sukhasana (no. 14) and Virasana (no. 15).

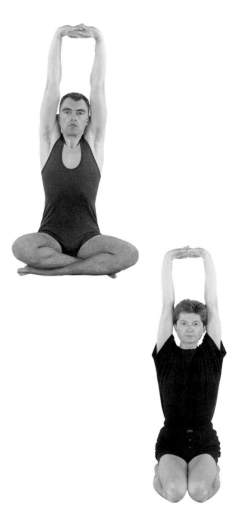

Interlock the fingers. Turn the palms away from you, stretch the arms forward and then up over the head. Do not arch the back at the waist. Tighten the elbows and stretch as much as you can.

Stay for 20–30 seconds, then bring the arms down. Change the interlock of the fingers (by placing the right ones in front of the left or vice versa) and repeat.

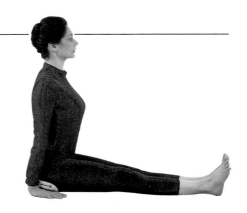

18 · DANDASANA
STAFF POSE

Sit on one or two blankets with the legs stretched straight in front of you. Tighten the knees and stretch the feet. Extend the heels and soles, and point the toes up.

Place the palms or fingertips beside the hips and press them down. Stretch the trunk up, paying special attention to lifting the lower back. Extend the spine up from the base. Open the chest to take the shoulders back. Keep the head straight. Relax the eyes and look straight ahead.

Stay for 20–30 seconds, then release.

19 · SIDDHASANA
PERFECT POSE

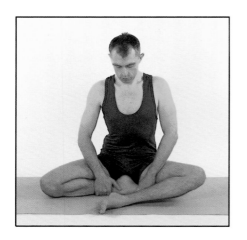

1 Sit in Dandasana (no. 18). Bend the right knee as far to the right as possible, hold the foot from underneath and bring it toward the pubis. Revolve the ankle so that the sole of the foot faces up.

2 Bend the left leg similarly to the left and place the heel on top of the right, sole face up. Tuck in the toes of the left foot between the right thigh and calf and the toes of the right foot between the left thigh and calf. Centre the feet in front of the pubis and open the thighs outward. Stretch the trunk up, especially the lower back. Place the hands on the knees and press them outward, without separating the feet. Maintain a firm posture, with the back straight.

Stay for 30–60 seconds, then change the legs.

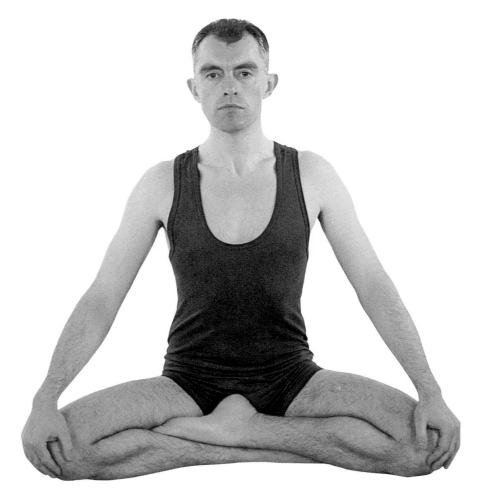

20 · GOMUKHASANA (ARMS ONLY)
HEAD-OF-COW POSE

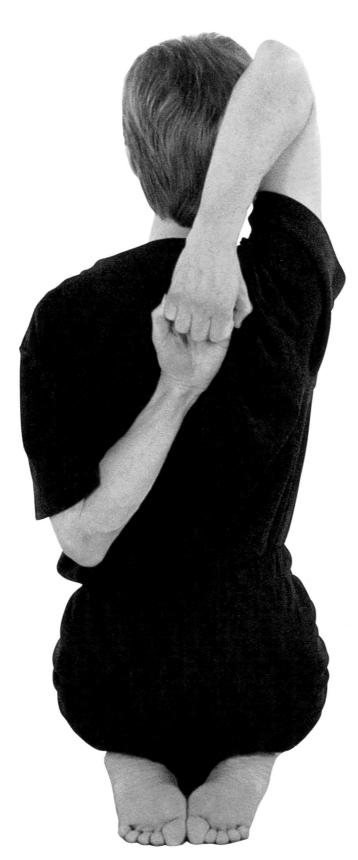

Left: Sit on the heels, or in Virasana (no. 15) or Sukhasana (no. 14). Bend the right arm behind the back, and stretch the hand and forearm up along the spine, with the palm facing out. Bring the elbow in with the other hand.

Stretch the left arm up, turn it so that the palm faces back, then bend the elbow and catch the right hand. Clasp the hands as far as possible. Take the right shoulder back and point the left elbow toward the ceiling. Keep the chest level.

Stay for 30–60 seconds, then repeat on the other side.

VARIANT (STANDING)

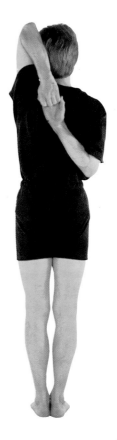

These arm movements can also be done while standing.

21 · JANUSIRSASANA

HEAD-TO-KNEE POSE

● *In case of lower back pain, do not practise the full pose.*

CONCAVE

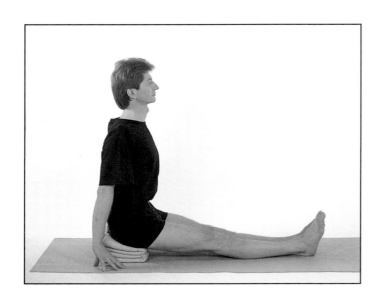

1 Sit in Dandasana (no. 18) on one or two folded blankets. If your lower back is stiff, you will need more height.

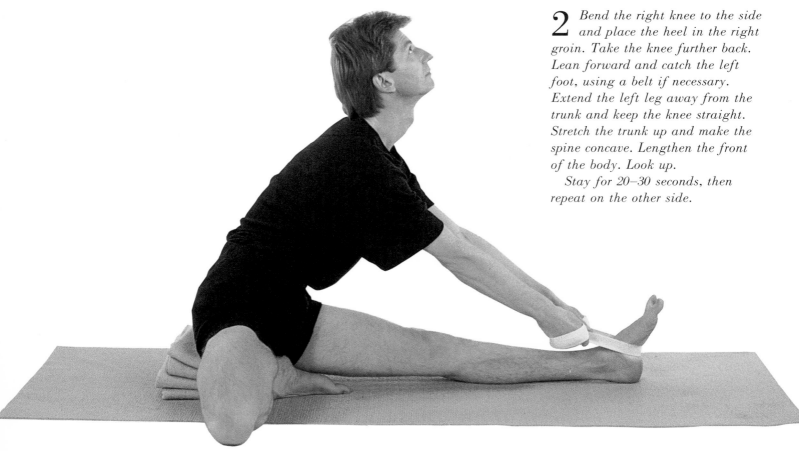

2 Bend the right knee to the side and place the heel in the right groin. Take the knee further back. Lean forward and catch the left foot, using a belt if necessary. Extend the left leg away from the trunk and keep the knee straight. Stretch the trunk up and make the spine concave. Lengthen the front of the body. Look up.
 Stay for 20–30 seconds, then repeat on the other side.

FULL POSE

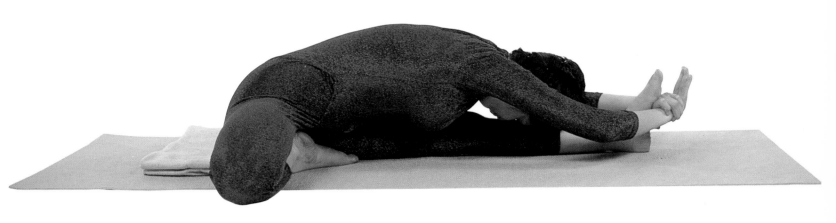

*Follow steps 1 and 2. With an
exhalation bend forward over the
left leg. Catch further and take the
head down to the shin.*
   *Stay for 20–30 seconds, then
repeat on the other side.*

*VARIANT (HEAD ON
BOLSTER)*

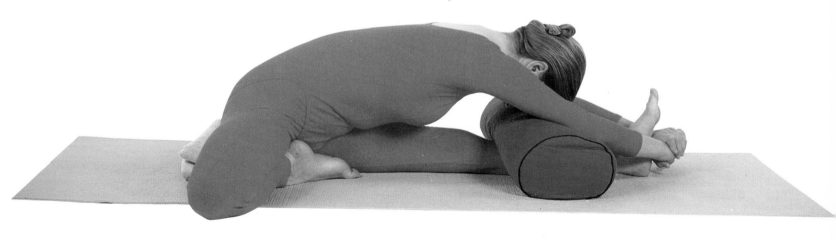

*Follow steps 1 and 2. Rest the head
on a folded blanket or bolster.*
   *Stay for 1–2 minutes, then repeat
on the other side.*

● *If you are stiff, rest the head on
a stool. If there is strain in the
knee, support it and reduce the
length of time in the posture.*

22 · TRIANG MUKHAIKAPADA PASCIMOTTANASANA
FORWARD BEND WITH ONE LEG BENT BACK

CONCAVE

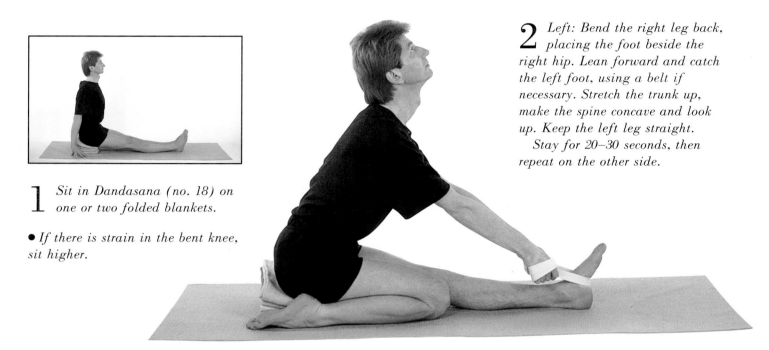

1 Sit in Dandasana (no. 18) on one or two folded blankets.

● If there is strain in the bent knee, sit higher.

2 Left: Bend the right leg back, placing the foot beside the right hip. Lean forward and catch the left foot, using a belt if necessary. Stretch the trunk up, make the spine concave and look up. Keep the left leg straight.
 Stay for 20–30 seconds, then repeat on the other side.

FULL POSE

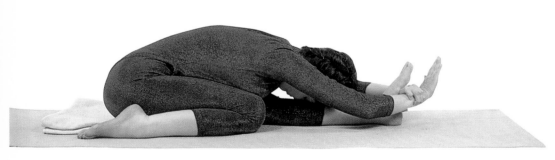

Follow steps 1 and 2 above. With an exhalation, bend forward over the left leg. Elongate the trunk and catch further. Take the head down.
 Stay for 20–30 seconds, then repeat on the other side.

VARIANT (HEAD ON BOLSTER)

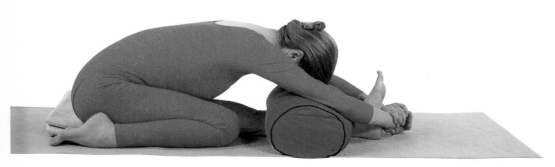

Follow steps 1 and 2 above. Rest the head on a blanket or bolster.
 Stay for 1–2 minutes, then repeat on the other side.

● If you are stiff, rest the head on a stool.

23 · MARICYASANA I (TWIST ONLY)

SIMPLE TWIST CATCHING THE ARMS BEHIND

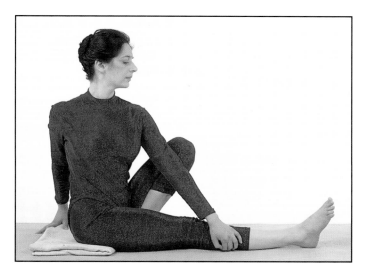

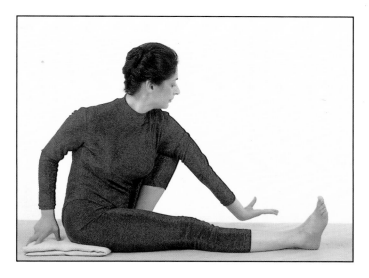

1 Sit in Dandasana (no. 18) on one or two folded blankets. Bend the left knee up and bring the foot in front of the pubis. Place the inner edge of the foot against the right inner thigh. Keep the right leg extended. Turn to the right, and bring the left upper arm in front of the left knee. Place the right hand beside the right hip.

2 Press the fingertips of the right hand into the floor, and the left arm against the left knee, to turn the trunk more. Rotate the left arm inward so that the palm faces back.

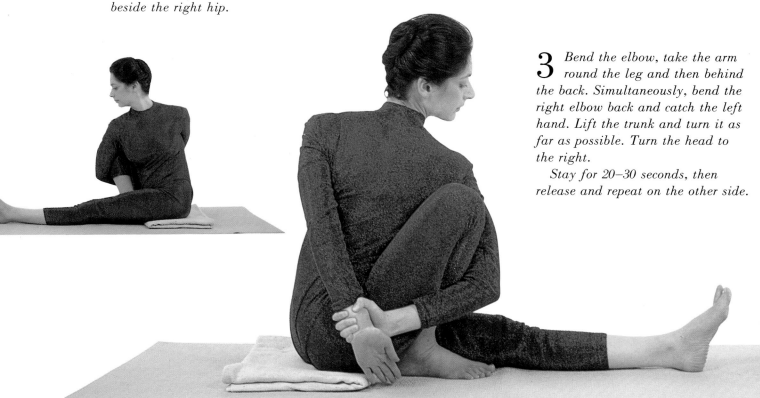

3 Bend the elbow, take the arm round the leg and then behind the back. Simultaneously, bend the right elbow back and catch the left hand. Lift the trunk and turn it as far as possible. Turn the head to the right.

Stay for 20–30 seconds, then release and repeat on the other side.

24 · PASCIMOTTANASANA
FULL FORWARD BEND

CONCAVE

FULL POSE

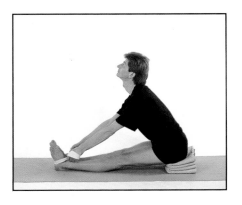

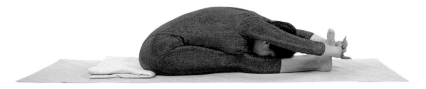

Follow the method as above, then bend forward over the legs, catching further with the hands. Stretch the front of the body and the spine to go further. Maintain an even extension of both legs and both sides of the body. Take the head down.

Stay for 20–30 seconds, then come up.

Sit in Dandasana (no. 18) on one or two folded blankets. Lean forward and catch the feet, using a belt if necessary. Stretch the trunk up. Make the back concave, lift the chest and look up. Keep the knees straight.

Stay for 20–30 seconds, then release.

VARIANT (HEAD ON BOLSTER)

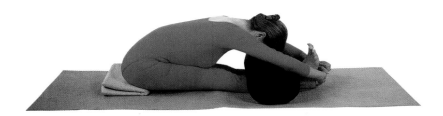

Do the posture as above, resting the head on a bolster or blankets.

Quieten the mind. Stay for 2–3 minutes, then come up.

25 · MALASANA (PREPARATORY)
GARLAND POSE

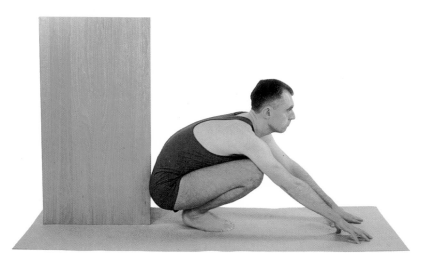

Squat, leaning the lower back against a wall. Keep the heels down if possible. Spread the knees apart but keep the feet together. Take the trunk down between the thighs and knees. Stretch the arms and chest forward, with the hands on the floor.

Stay for 30–60 seconds, then stand up.

SUPINE AND PRONE POSES

26 · CROSS BOLSTERS

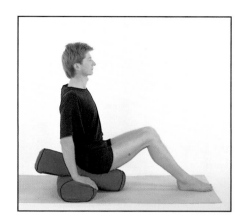

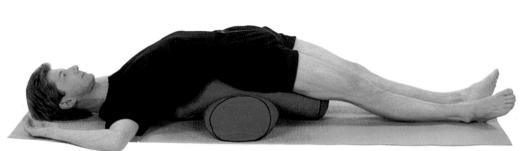

1 *Arrange two bolsters as a cross on the floor, with the lengthwise one on top. Sit on the bolsters.*

2 *Lie back and stretch the legs forward. Place the lower back on the highest part of the bolster arrangement and the shoulders on the floor. You can tie the thighs together with a belt for a passive extension and to make the posture more restful. Take the arms over the* head *and relax. If the lower back feels pinched, pass the hands underneath it from waist to buttocks to lengthen and ease it.*

Stay for 3–5 minutes. To get up, slide back a little toward the head, then bend the knees and turn to the side.

27 · MATSYASANA (SIMPLE)

FISH POSE

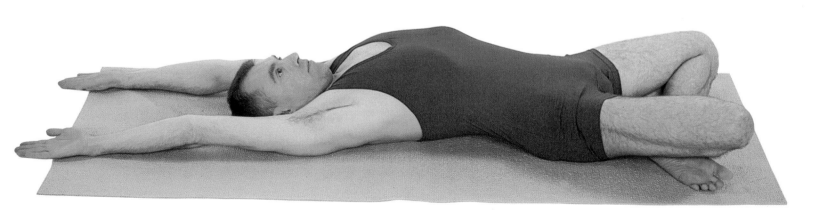

Sit in Sukhasana (no. 14). Lean back and lie down. While lying down, extend the lower back. Take the arms over the head and straighten the elbows. Stretch the whole trunk, especially the abdominal area.

Stay for 1–2 minutes, then come up, change the cross-legs and repeat.

28 · SUPTA BADDHAKONASANA
LYING DOWN IN BADDHAKONASANA

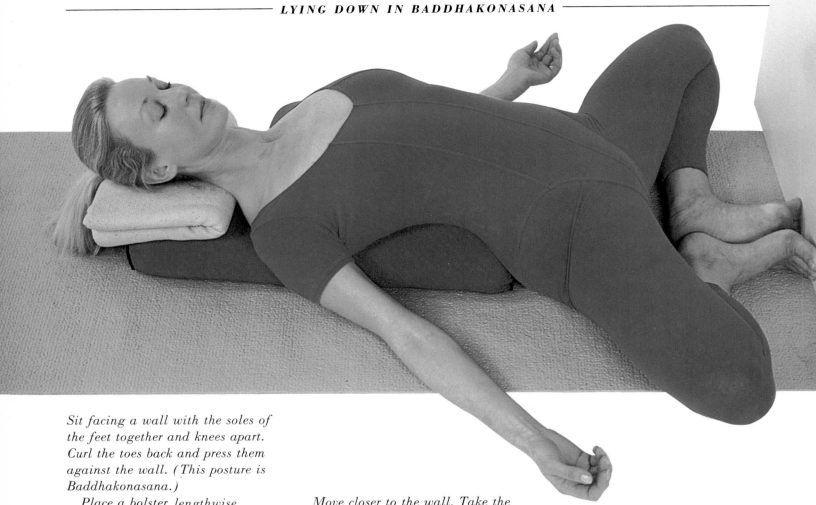

Sit facing a wall with the soles of
the feet together and knees apart.
Curl the toes back and press them
against the wall. (This posture is
Baddhakonasana.)

Place a bolster lengthwise
behind the lower back, hold it
toward you and lie back over it,
with the shoulders on the ground.

Move closer to the wall. Take the
arms over the head. Breathe evenly.
Stay for 2–5 minutes. Turn to the
side to get up.

• If your legs are uncomfortable,
place a blanket under the thighs.

29 · SUPTA VIRASANA
RECLINING HERO POSE

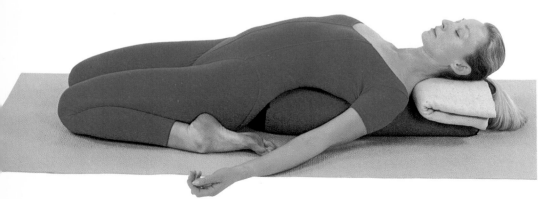

Sit in Virasana (no. 15). Place a
bolster (or folded blankets) behind
you. Hold it against the lower back
and lie down. Place an extra
blanket under the head if necessary.
Relax. Stay for 3–5 minutes, then
get up.

• If you need to sit on something in
Virasana you will also need a high
support under the back.

30 · *URDHVA PRASARITA PADASANA*

LEGS STRETCHED TO 90°

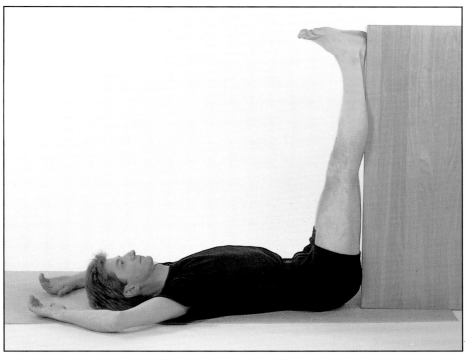

1 *Sit sideways to a wall and move the buttocks as close as possible to it. Take the legs up one at a time and swivel the body round. Lie down and rest the legs vertically against the wall. Take the arms over the head and relax.*

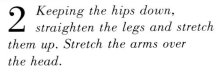

2 *Keeping the hips down, straighten the legs and stretch them up. Stretch the arms over the head.*
   Stay for 20–30 seconds (or longer). To come down, bend the knees and turn to the side.

31 · ADHO MUKHA SVANASANA
──── DOG POSE ────

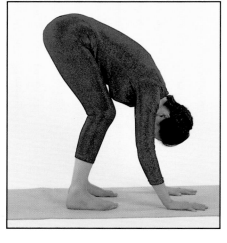

2 *Below: Step about 3–4 ft (90–120 cm) back and straighten the legs, so that the body makes an inverted "V" shape. Lift up the hips, press the thighs back and extend the heels downward.*

Straighten the elbows, lift the shoulders and stretch the trunk up. Keep the arms and legs firm. Relax the head.

Stay for 20–30 seconds, then bend the knees and come down.

1 *Stand in Tadasana (no. 1). Take the feet hip-width apart. Bend down and place the palms on the floor in front of the feet and shoulder-width apart. Spread the fingers.*

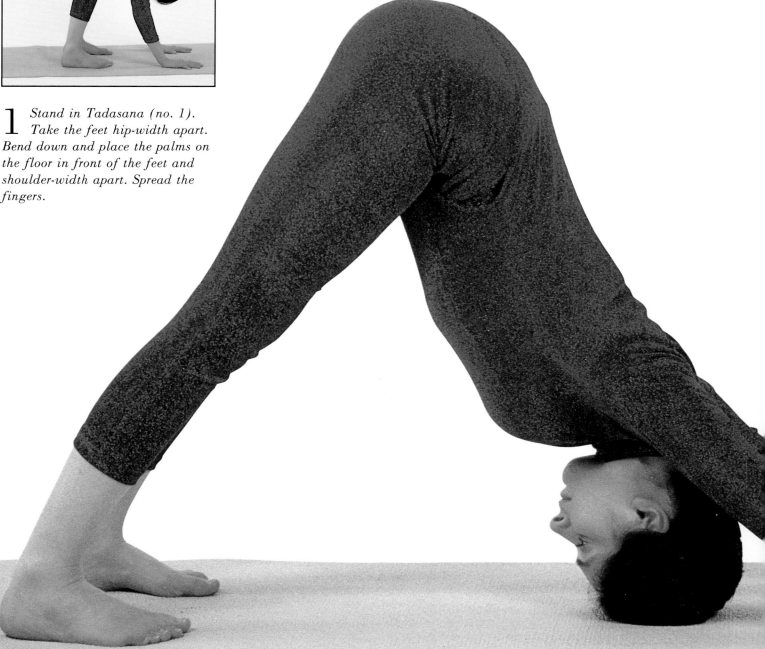

VARIANT (HEAD SUPPORTED)

1 *Right: Place a folded blanket or bolster lengthwise a short distance from the wall. Kneel in front of it. Place the hands, palms down, near the wall. Touch the wall with the thumbs and index fingers, spreading them as far apart as possible.*

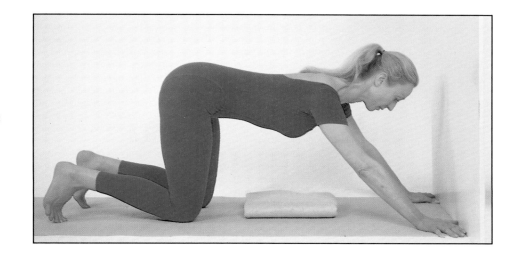

2 *Below: Raise the hips and straighten the legs. Rest the head on the blanket. Stretch the arms and trunk up strongly. Do not let the weight of the body sink on to the head. Relax the head.*
  Stay for 30–60 seconds, then come down.

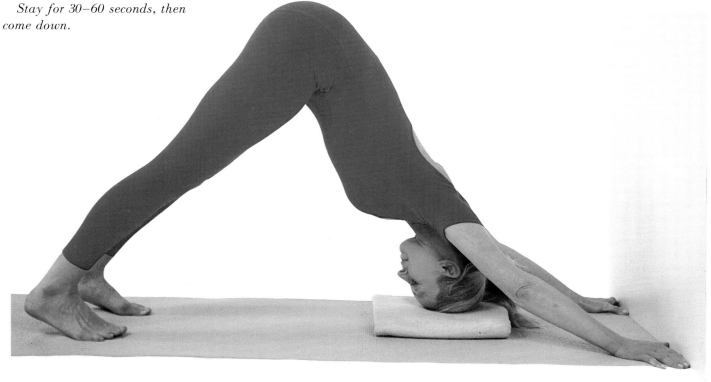

TWISTING POSES

32 · MARICYASANA (STANDING)
——— STANDING TWIST ———

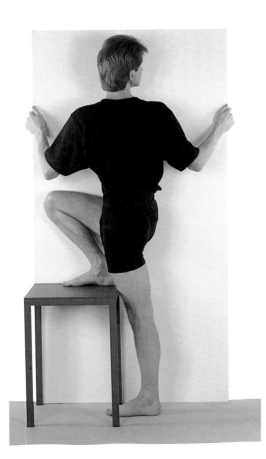

Place a high stool or small table
near a wall or ledge. Stand in
Tadasana (no. 1) with the right
side of the body by the wall. Raise
the right foot on to the stool and
press the foot down. Keep the right
thigh touching the wall. Stretch the
trunk up and turn toward the wall,
holding on with the hands wherever
possible to give you leverage. Keep
the left leg and trunk vertical, and
the foot facing forward. Turn as
far as you can.

Stay for 20–30 seconds, come
down and repeat on the other side.

33 · BHARADVAJASANA
——— SIMPLE TWIST ———

PREPARATORY

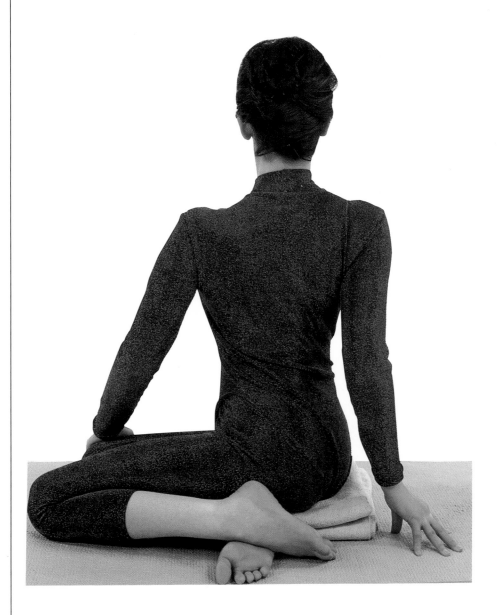

Sit in Dandasana (no. 18) on
one or two folded blankets. Bend
the legs to the left. Place the
left foot on top of the right
instep, with the sole of the left
foot facing up. Extend the spine
and the trunk up. Turn to the
right. Place the left hand on the
outer side of the right knee and
the right hand beside the right
hip. Use the arms to help turn
the trunk. Turn the hips, waist
and chest as far as you can.

Stay for 20–30 seconds. Turn
to the front, and repeat on the
other side.

FULL POSE

VARIANT (ON A CHAIR)

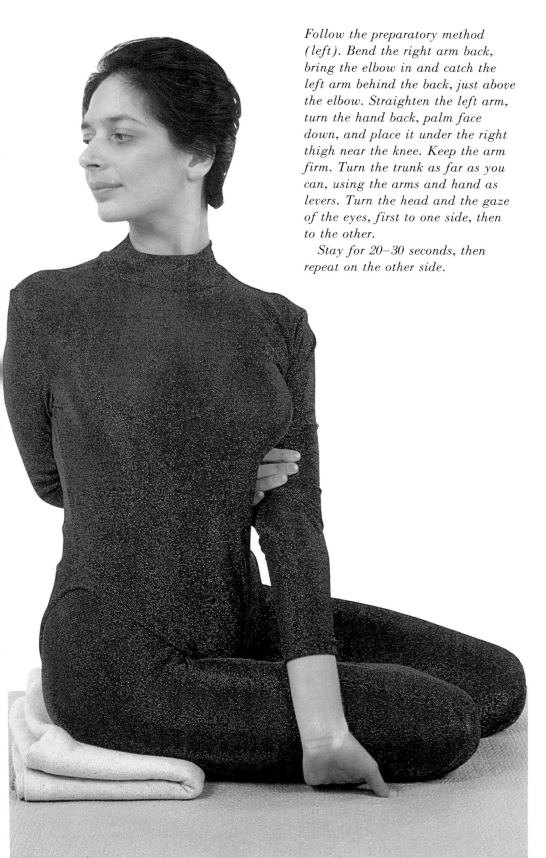

Follow the preparatory method (left). Bend the right arm back, bring the elbow in and catch the left arm behind the back, just above the elbow. Straighten the left arm, turn the hand back, palm face down, and place it under the right thigh near the knee. Keep the arm firm. Turn the trunk as far as you can, using the arms and hand as levers. Turn the head and the gaze of the eyes, first to one side, then to the other.

Stay for 20–30 seconds, then repeat on the other side.

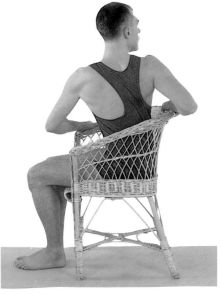

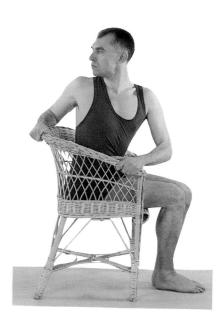

Sit on a chair, with the knees and feet together. Lift the hips, waist and ribcage. Turn to the right, holding the back of the chair. Keep the trunk vertical and lifted and turn to the maximum. Turn the head and neck to the right.

Stay for 20–30 seconds, then repeat on the other side.

INVERTED POSES

34 · SARVANGASANA
—— NECK BALANCE ——

1 *Prepare a set of four or five folded blankets, with the folded edges neatly together. The height should be 2–3 inches (5–7.5 cm), the width sufficient for the shoulders, and the depth enough to accommodate the length of the upper arms. If the arms and elbows slip apart, tie a belt round the upper arms, just above the elbows, approximately shoulder width apart.*

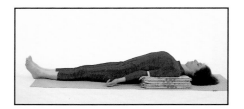

Lie down with the shoulders on the blankets, 2–3 inches (5–7.5 cm) away from the edge, and the head on the floor. Check that you are in a straight line.

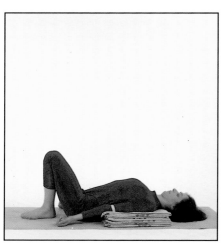

2 *Flex the knees and bring the feet toward the buttocks. Then lift the lower back slightly and lengthen it away from you.*

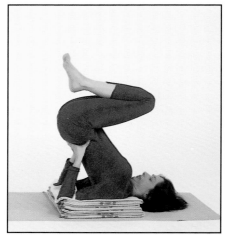

3 *Bend the knees over the abdomen and swing the trunk and the legs up. Immediately support the back with your hands and open the chest.*

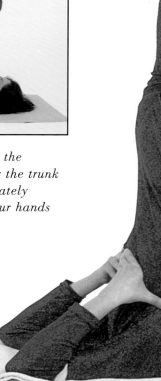

4 *Straighten the legs up. Move the hands further up the back towards the shoulder blades to give you maximum lift and support. Bring the chest toward the chin. Stretch the whole body up. Keep the posture stable.*

    Stay for 2–5 minutes. To come down, bend the legs and slide down.

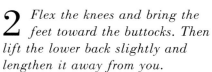

35 · HALASANA
PLOUGH POSE

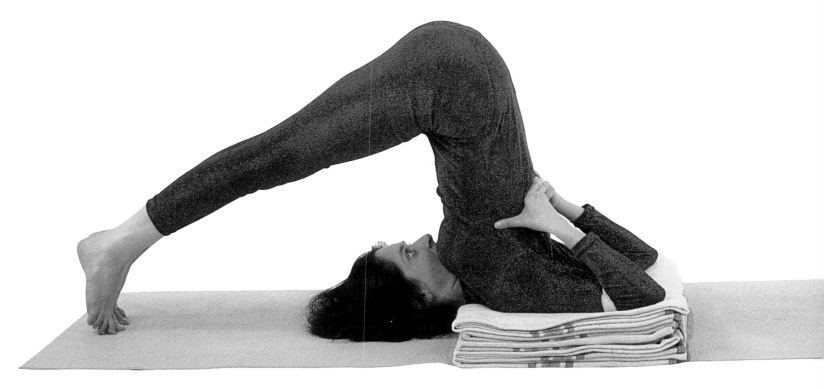

=== NOTE ===

● Inverted poses should not be practised during menstruation.
● If you experience pressure in the head, eyes, ears or throat in any inverted pose, come down and rest. Then seek advice.

From Sarvangasana (no. 34) take the legs down over the head and rest the feet on the floor. Keep the hands on the back, lift the trunk and extend front of the body up. Straighten the knees and stretch the legs away from the hips. Relax the face, the eyes and the ears.

Stay for 2–5 minutes, then slide down.

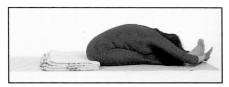

● *If you wish, after sliding down from Halasana, sit on the edge of the blanket and rest forward in Pascimottanasana (no. 24).*

36 · ARDHA HALASANA
HALF PLOUGH POSE

Place a chair or stool over the head before you go up into Sarvangasana (no. 34). From Sarvangasana take the legs down on to the chair to support the thighs.

Take the arms over the head and relax. Do not let the shoulders slip off the blankets.

Stay for 3–5 minutes. Come down with bent knees and ease yourself off the stool, at the same time pushing it away with the hands. Slide down.

● *If you have a long trunk you may increase the height by placing a bolster or blankets on the stool.*
● *If your back is very stiff, keep the stool further away and support the shins.*
● *If the neck hurts, increase the height of the blankets.*

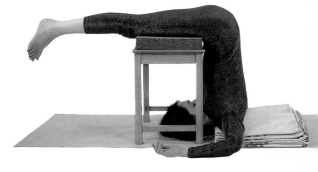

37 · SARVANGASANA (ON CHAIR)

NECK BALANCE

Use a sturdy armchair that will not topple. Take each stage slowly and carefully, so that you feel secure.

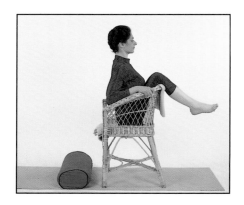

1 *Place a bolster crosswise on the floor in front of the armchair. Sit facing the back of the chair, with the legs bent over the back of it and holding on to the sides.*

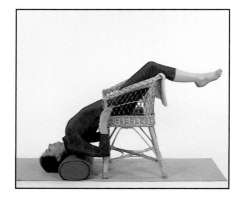

3 *Lean back further so that the waist curves over the edge of the seat and the head goes down.*

4 *Below: Rest the shoulders on the bolster. Straighten the legs and stretch them against the back of the chair. Depending on the construction of the chair, hold the chair or take the arms over the head. Keep the back ribs tucked in and the chest open.*

Stay for 5–8 minutes, then come down as shown in steps 5–7.

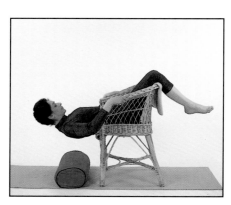

2 *Move the hips closer to the back of the chair, hold the arms and lean back.*

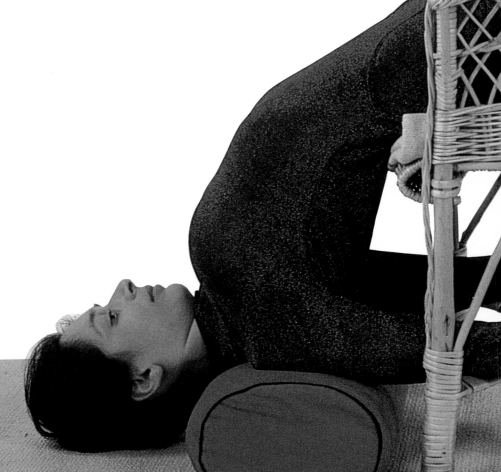

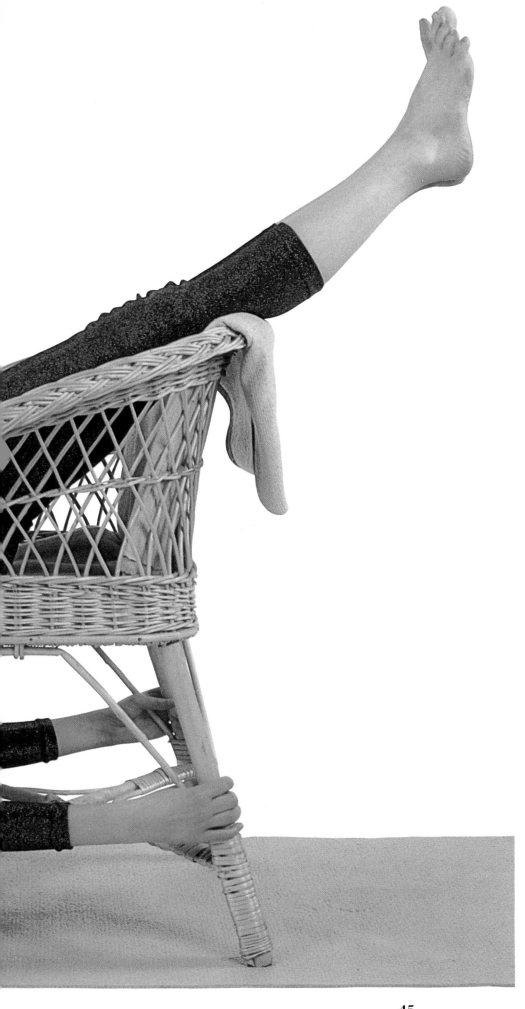

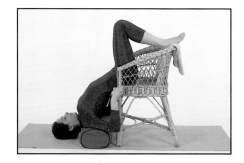

5 Bend the legs and place the feet on the back of the armchair. Hold the arms of the chair.

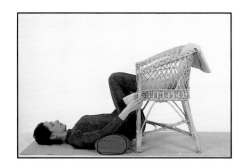

6 Slide backward off the armchair till the lower back rests on the bolster. Stay for a moment.

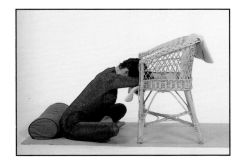

7 Turn to the side, sit cross-legged in front of the chair and rest your head on it.

You may need to experiment with bolsters and blankets to obtain the height you need.

38 · SARVANGASANA (AGAINST WALL)

NECK BALANCE AGAINST WALL

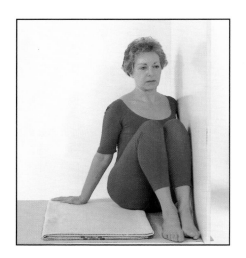

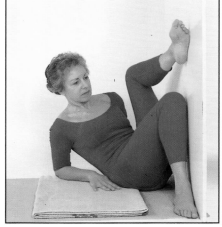

5 *Below: Support the back with the hands and bring the elbows in. Straighten the legs, keeping the feet on the wall. Lift the chest, abdomen and hips. Breathe evenly. Stay for 3–5 minutes, then bend the legs and come down.*

1 *Place one or two folded blankets near a wall, with the folded edges away from it. Sit on them sideways, as close to the wall as possible.*

2 *Lean back on to the elbows, swivel the trunk round and take one leg up the wall.*

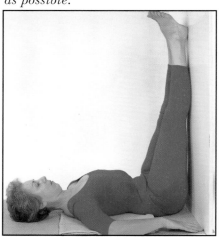

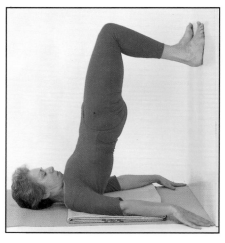

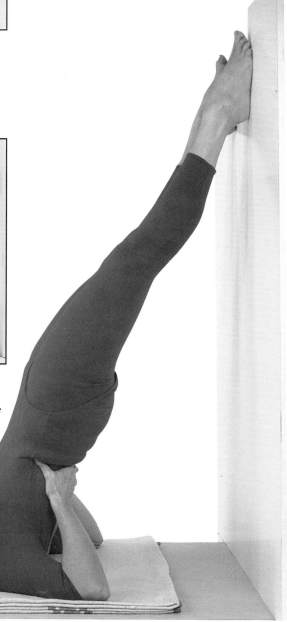

3 *Take the other leg up the wall and lie back. Place the buttocks against the wall, the shoulders on the blankets, and the head on the floor.*

4 *Bend the legs, press the feet against the wall and raise the hips and chest.*

39 · SETU BANDHA SARVANGASANA (SUPPORTED)
─── NECK BALANCE BACK ARCH ───

This posture may be done during menstruation. To make the pose more restful, tie a belt round the middle thighs.

ON BOLSTER

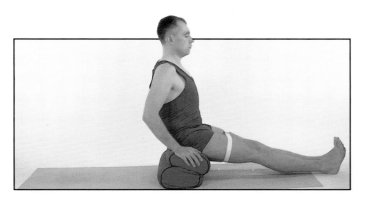

1 Place two bolsters on top of each other horizontally on the floor and sit on them.

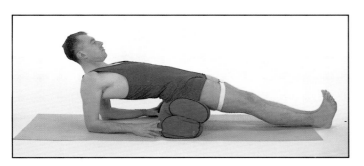

2 Slide slightly back so that the lower back is nearly off the bolster.

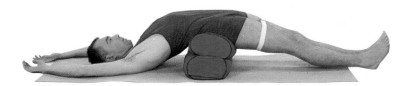

3 Support yourself on your arms. Lie back with the shoulders and head on the floor. Take the arms over the head and relax. Stay for 5–8 minutes.

● If the lower back feels pinched, stretch it away from the waist or raise the feet and support them.
● To come down, bend the knees, push the bolsters away and slide back. Remove the belt (if used). Turn to the side, then sit cross-legged in front of the bolsters and bend forward, resting the head on them.

ON BENCH

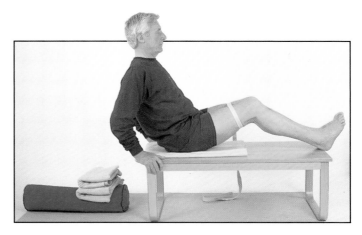

1 Place one or two blankets on a sturdy bench. Place a bolster lengthwise on the floor in front of it. Sit backwards near the edge of the bench and take the feet up on to it.

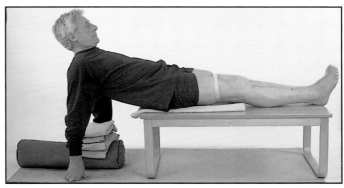

2 Place the hands on the floor. Lean back, curving the waist over the edge of the bench. Straighten the legs.

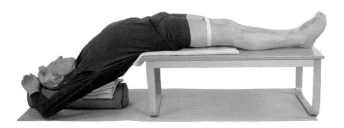

3 Rest the shoulders and head on the bolster. Take the arms over the head. Stay for 5–8 minutes.

40 · VIPARITA KARANI
RESTFUL INVERSION

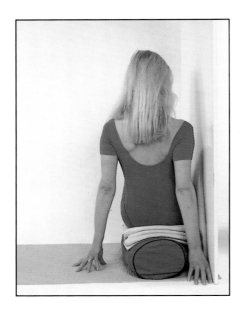 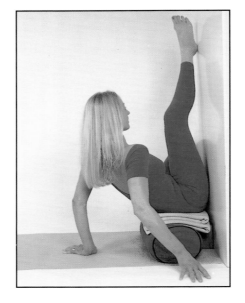

1 *Place a block or thick book against the wall, with a bolster in front of it. Place one or more folded blankets on top, depending on your height. Sit sideways on the bolster, with the right hip touching the wall.*

2 *With the help of the hands, swivel the body round and take the right leg up the wall. Keep the right buttock against the wall.*

3 *Continue to swivel the body round and take the left leg up. At the same time lean back till the shoulders and head reach the floor. Support the lower back on the bolster arrangement and rest the buttocks and legs against the wall. Take the arms over the head and relax.*

Stay for 5-8 minutes. Bend the knees, slide back, turn to the side and get up.

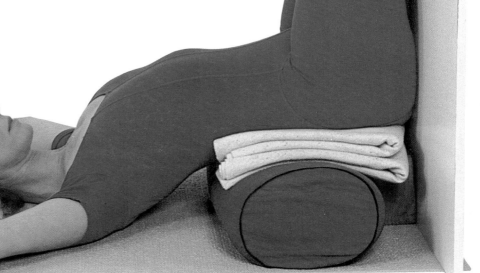

RELAXATION

41 · SAVASANA

CORPSE POSE

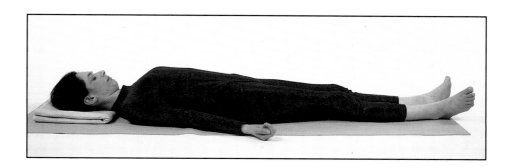

Lie on the floor in a straight line, with the feet together. Line yourself up carefully, as any lack of alignment prevents you from relaxing completely. Stretch the arms and legs and then relax them. Keep the arms slightly away from the trunk, with the palms facing up. Allow the legs and feet to roll away from each other.

    Place a blanket under the head and neck at a comfortable height, so that the forehead and chin do not tilt backward. Close the eyes

and let go mentally. Observe whether you are lying evenly on the floor. Feel the weight of the body sinking into the floor and the mind

becoming quiet. Breathe evenly.
    Stay for 5–10 minutes. To get up, slowly open the eyes, bend the knees and turn to the side.

VARIANT (ON A BOLSTER)

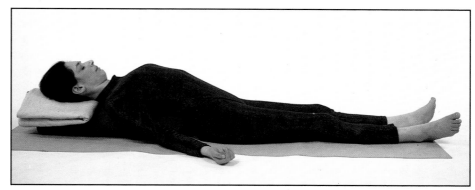

Place a bolster or two narrowly folded blankets lengthwise on the floor. Sit in front of the bolster and hold it against your back. Lean back and lie down on it. Centre the spine on it. Place a folded blanket under the head. Press the shoulders down and away from the neck. Move the back of the head away from the shoulders. Stretch the arms and legs away from the trunk and then relax them. Relax the hands and fingers, palms face up. Extend the soles of the feet and the toes, then let the feet drop to the sides.

Close the eyes and relax. Breathe quietly and enjoy the feeling of the chest opening with the support of the bolster.

Stay for 5–10 minutes. Before getting up slowly open the eyes, bend the knees and turn to the side.

When Savasana is done on a bolster, the mind and body relax well as the chest is open, and breathing comes easily. The posture strengthens the lungs and is thus a good preparation for pranayama.

TOWARD MENTAL PEACE

Pranayama is control of the breath, from the subtlest to the most complex level. According to Patanjali it is not to be attempted until practice of the postures is mastered and, according to orthodox tradition, it is not to be attempted except under expert supervision.

The purpose of the postures and breathing exercises is the development of a sound and healthy body and mind. Yoga philosophy insists that this must be achieved before a person can embark on a programme of philosophical and spiritual development.

Without the one, the other is not possible. But when the foundation is firm, progress is assured.

RELAXING THE BODY

Lie on a bolster in Savasana (no. 41, variant). Spend a few minutes relaxing the body. Release tension from the feet and legs, the arms and hands, the abdomen and the face. Still your thoughts.

Keep the eyes quiet. Let the eyeballs sink down into the eye-sockets. Relax the temples and the forehead. Relax the skin at the bridge of the nose. Relax the cheeks by releasing them away from the eyes. Relax the jaws, moving the lower jaw a little away from the upper, without tensing it. Quieten the ears. Feel the connection between the ear passages and the jaws and relax them. Keep the tongue still. Let it rest on the lower palate and as it relaxes, allow the root of the tongue to recede into the throat. Do not clench the teeth; keep them very slightly parted.

Relax the neck and throat. If you cannot relax them, press the shoulders down and move the shoulder-blades into the back ribs. At the same time bring the chin slightly down towards the throat. Quieten the vibrations of the vocal cords.

In the early stages of your practice, end your relaxation here. Lie flat on your back, then bend the legs and turn to the side before getting up.

OBSERVING THE BREATH

Spend about five minutes relaxing on a bolster as described above.

When the body feels relaxed, begin to observe your breathing. Take the gaze of the eyes downward and then inward into the chest. Follow the course of the breath. Do not alter it, but watch the rhythm of your normal breathing. Observe whether you are breathing evenly and equally in both nostrils. Observe the speed of the breath, and whether your inhalations and exhalations are the same length. Keep your breathing soft and quiet.

Continue in the same way for a few minutes. As you watch the breath, do not lose the awareness of your relaxation. Maintain the quiet state of the body from moment to moment.

Relaxation needs to be learned. You will find that while you are concentrating on the breath,

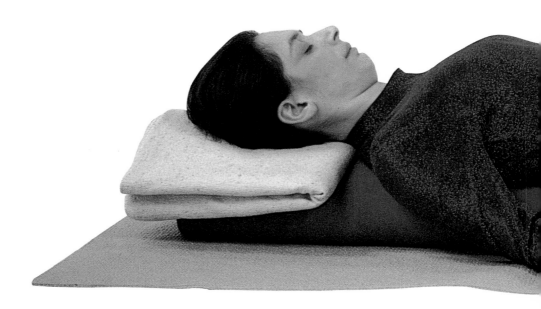

tension creeps into different parts of the body. Some areas of tension are common to everyone. During inhalation, everyone has the habit of moving the head backward and lifting the chin; move them back to their original position every time. Similarly, tension returns unconsciously to the hands and feet, and the abdomen. Release this tension as soon as you observe it, during exhalation.

Other areas of tension in the body are individual, depending on each person's physique and habitual posture. Injuries, stiffness and the asymmetrical development of muscles and joints all prevent the free flow of energy and relaxation in the body. So too do mental and emotional strain. This is why the practice of postures is necessary: they counteract the wear and tear of daily life.

Relaxation and pranayama go one step further by training the mind to look inward. They induce a state of calmness that can be experienced again and again. This develops a reserve of inner strength.

The next stage of your relaxation can end here for the first few weeks of practice. When you have gained more experience you may continue by deeping your relaxation (see overleaf).

PREPARATORY PRANAYAMA TEN-WEEK COURSE

Sundays in the ten-week course are devoted to relaxing poses. Pranayama preparation can be added to these in the following way:

WEEKS 1 & 2   *Relaxing the Body*

WEEKS 3 & 4   *Observing the Breath*

WEEK 5   **Repeat weeks 1–4**

WEEKS 6 & 7   *Deepening your Relaxation*
Add: *Normal Inhalation, Lengthened Exhalation* and *Lengthened Inhalation, Normal Inhalation*

WEEKS 8 & 9   *Deepening your Relaxation*
Add: *Lengthened Inhalation and Exhalation*

WEEK 10   **Repeat any of the techniques given in weeks 6–9.**

Below: For relaxation practice, lie on a bolster in Savasana (no. 41, variant), opening the chest well. Ensure that you are settled comfortably so there is no physical distraction from your relaxation.

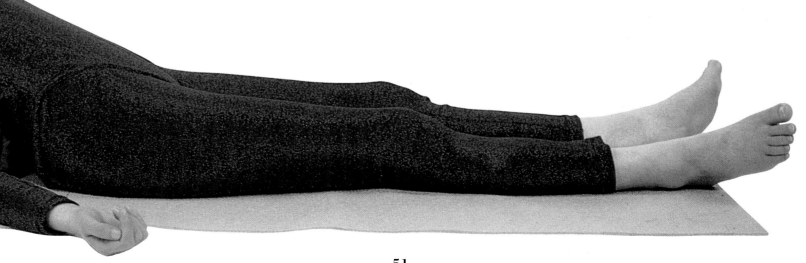

DEEPENING RELAXATION

After spending a few minutes observing your normal breathing, practise the following technique for lengthening the breath.

Normal Inhalation, Lengthened Exhalation

First exhale and relax the abdomen. Inhale normally. Exhale slowly and quietly. Do not strain. Again take a normal inhalation, then exhale slowly and quietly.

Continue in this way for about five minutes. Then lie quietly and breathe normally. Enjoy lying down and relaxing. Allow a few minutes to elapse before continuing.

Lengthened Inhalation, Normal Exhalation

Exhale completely, then take a slow, quiet inhalation. Do not breathe in suddenly or deeply, but lengthen the breath smoothly. Exhale normally. Again inhale slowly and quietly, taking care not to tense the eyes or brain. Do not let the breath disturb the nostrils. Exhale normally.

Continue in this way for about five minutes. Then lie quietly and breathe normally.

Allow a few minutes to elapse before continuing.

This is enough breathing practice for the first few sessions.

Lengthened Inhalations and Exhalations

Exhale completely, to empty the lungs of stale air and to prepare yourself psychologically. Inhale slowly and quietly, lengthening the breath as above. Do not hurry. Then exhale slowly and softly, lengthening the breath as above. Relax completely. Again take a quiet, slow inhalation, without tensing, and then a quiet, slow exhalation.

Continue for about five minutes, then breathe normally.

ENDING YOUR RELAXATION

Bend the legs, turn to the side, remove the bolster from under you, and lie flat on the back in Savasana. Keep the blanket for the head. Settle down on the floor; keep the mind quiet. Let go completely. Relax the brain. Move the awareness down into the chest.

Then carefully open the eyes, bend the knees and turn to the right side. Stay for a little while, then turn to the left. Get up from the side, or from the front.

Below: Savasana (no. 41) without a bolster is used for the final stage of relaxation practice. Check that your body is in alignment and lie still, keeping the mind and body quiet.

CONCLUSION

If Patanjali's teachings are followed and the inner body and the mind and nervous system are strengthened through asana practice, then the beginning stages of pranayama may safely be practised. However, it is preferable to have an experienced teacher to guide you in the early stages. Traditionally, it was considered essential to have a guru.

Until relaxation is learnt thoroughly, and the lungs are trained to alter their breathing pattern without strain, pranayama, the control of the breath, cannot be learnt. This is why, traditionally, it is not taught to beginners. One yoga text says that learning to control the breath is like learning to tame a tiger. The "father" of yoga, Patanjali, says that the practice of asanas must be mastered first.

The explanations of yoga in this book are aimed to be a guide to the first steps of yoga practice. The end of yoga is meditation and spiritual awareness. These refined mental and spiritual states cannot be experienced without due preparation. The path is acknowledged to be long, but the benefits at every step are so great that countless people, of former ages and today, have found the effort worthwhile.

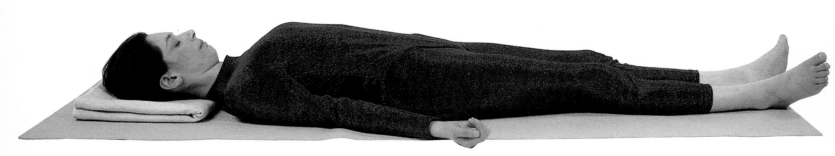

TOOLS FOR PRACTICE

In the Iyengar method props and equipment are used in yoga practice when the body cannot achieve a posture or make a particular effort to achieve a required result of its own accord. This principle is important in yoga therapy, but is also useful when practising generally.

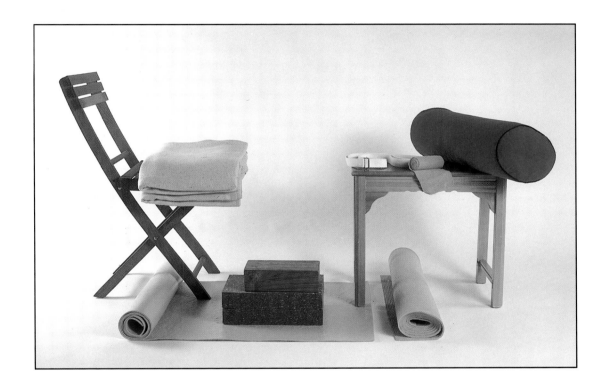

Most of the items required are common equipment found in a home. If the exact "prop" is not available, it can usually be substituted by something else.

Supporting the body in the asanas enables muscular extensions to be done in a passive way. It also helps to improve blood circulation and respiratory capacity.

The items used in this book are:

● **Armchair** For supported Sarvangasana (no. 37).
● **Bandage** In forward bends, to wind round the forehead.
● **Belt** In Sarvangasana (no. 34), to keep the elbows in.
In forward bends, to help catch the foot.
● **Bench** For Setu Bandha Sarvangasana (no. 39) to arch the back and open the chest.
● **Blankets** For Sarvangasana (no. 34) and Halasana (no. 35), to prevent compression of the neck.

For sitting poses, to lift the lower back.
For Savasana (no. 41), to support the head.
● **Block/Brick** In standing poses, to support the lower hand when it is difficult to reach the floor.
● **Bolsters** In supine poses, to support the back and lift the chest.
● **Chair** In twists, to facilitate the turning of the spine to the maximum.
● **Door Post** For Supta Padangusthasana, to support the raised leg.

● **Ledge** In standing poses and twists, to allow an effective grip, enabling the body to turn.
● **Non-slip Mat** To prevent slipping in standing poses, etc.
● **Pole** In Uttanasana (no. 9), to increase the shoulder movement.
● **Stool** In Ardha Halasana (no. 36), to support the thighs for a restful pose.
In standing twists and leg raisings, to support the lifted leg.
● **Wall** In standing poses and twists, to give support and a sense of direction.

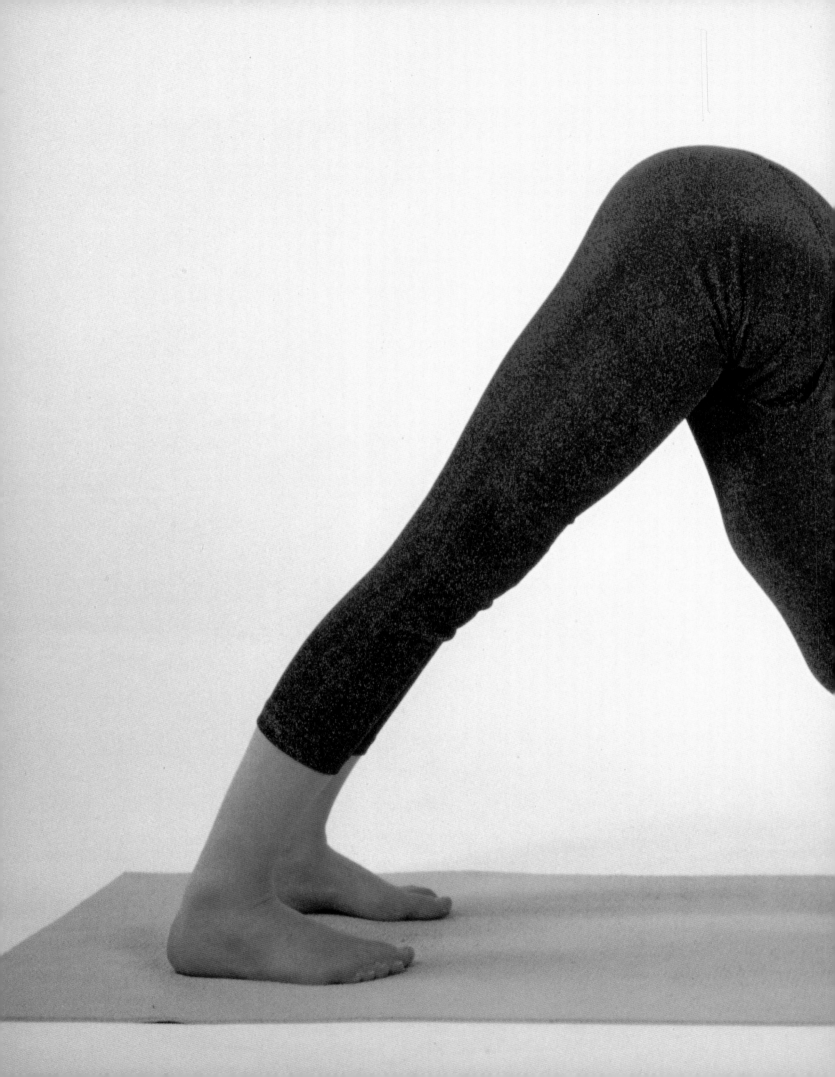

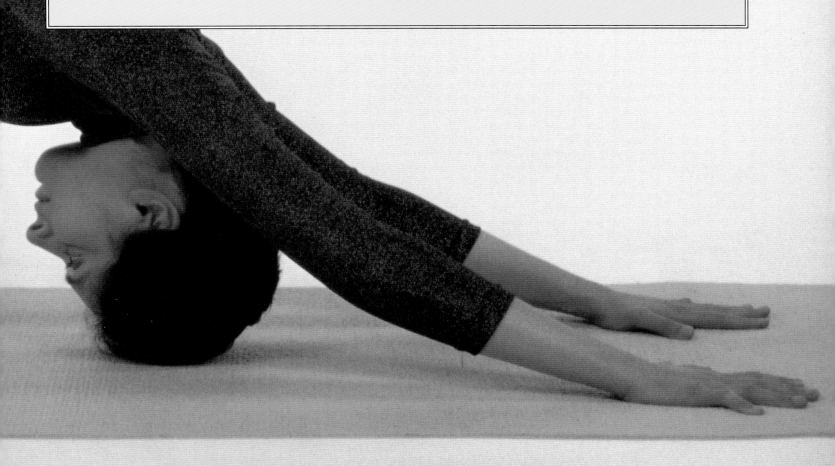

TEN-WEEK COURSE

The Asanas have been grouped according to the positioning of the body – standing, sitting, twisting, prone, supine, inverted and balancing – and your yoga practice may be structured so that different types of postures are incorporated into a single session. This course is devised for daily practice but it can be adapted to your own needs.

TEN-WEEK COURSE

The course consists of 41 postures (asanas) and their variants. Dynamic and relaxing poses are given on alternate days so that the body experiences a balance of effort and recuperation. As strength, stamina and suppleness increase, more postures are added.

The course is intended only as a guide to structuring your practice. Basic instructions for the postures are given in the Asana section. If at all possible, it is advisable to attend a class with a teacher as well as following the course.

The course is devised for daily practice, of approximately 30 minutes to one hour each day. It can be adapted or spread out according to individual need and circumstances.

The number of the postures refer to their sequence in the Asana section, an asterisk indicates that a posture is being introduced for the first time.

WEEK 1

MONDAY

*1 · *Tadasana*
*2 · *Vrksasana*
*3 · *Trikonasana*
*4 · *Parsvakonasana*
*6 · *Virabhadrasana II*
*9 · *Uttanasana* (on ledge)
*16 · *Virasana* (forward bend)
*14 · *Sukhasana*
*41 · *Savasana*

TUESDAY AND THURSDAY

9 · *Uttanasana* (on ledge)
*31 · *Adho Mukha Svanasana* (head supported)
14 · *Sukhasana*
*17 · *Parvatasana* (in Sukhasana)
*20 · *Gomukhasana* (arms only)
*39 · *Setu Bandha Sarvangasana* (on bolster)
*40 · *Viparita Karani*
41 · *Savasana*

WEDNESDAY AND FRIDAY

1 · *Tadasana*
2 · *Vrksasana*
3 · *Trikonasana*
4 · *Parsvakonasana*
6 · *Virabhadrasana II*
9 · *Uttanasana* (on ledge)
16 · *Virasana* (forward bend)
14 · *Sukhasana*
*34 · *Sarvangasana*
41 · *Savasana*

SATURDAY

1 · *Tadasana*
2 · *Vrksasana*
3 · *Trikonasana*
4 · *Parsvakonasana*
6 · *Virabhadrasana II*
9 · *Uttanasana* (on ledge)
16 · *Virasana* (forward bend)
*15 · *Virasana*
14 · *Sukhasana*
17 · *Parvatasana* (in Sukhasana)
20 · *Gomukhasana*
34 · *Sarvangasana*
*36 · *Ardha Halasana*
41 · *Savasana*

SUNDAY

*26 · *Cross Bolsters*
*27 · *Matsyasana* (simple)
31 · *Adho Mukha Svanasana* (head supported)
*9 · *Uttanasana*
39 · *Setu Bandha Sarvangasana* (on bolster)
40 · *Viparita Karani*
*41 · *Savasana* (on bolster)

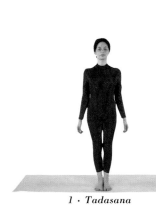

1 · *Tadasana*

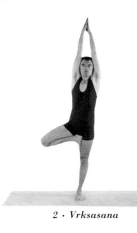

2 · *Vrksasana*

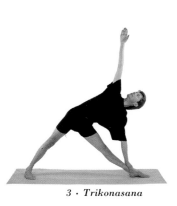

3 · *Trikonasana*

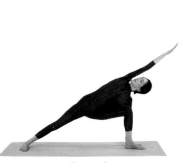

4 · *Parsvakonasana*

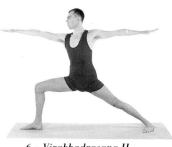

6 · Virabhadrasana II

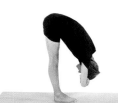

9 · Uttanasana

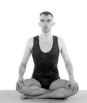

*9 · Uttanasana
(on ledge)*

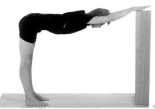

14 · Sukhasana

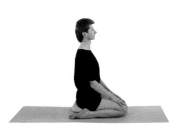

15 · Virasana

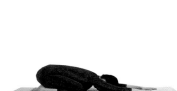

*16 · Virasana
(forward bend)*

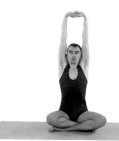

*17 · Parvatasana
(in Sukhasana)*

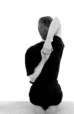

20 · Gomukhasana

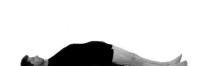

26 · Cross Bolsters

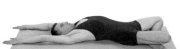

27 · Matsyasana

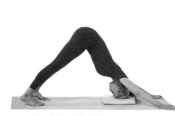

*31 · Adho Mukha
Svanasana (head supported)*

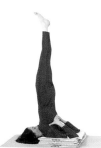

34 · Sarvangasana

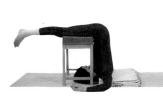

36 · Ardha Halasana

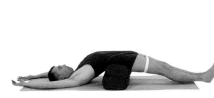

*39 · Setu Bandha Sarvangasana
(on bolster)*

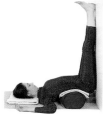

40 · Viparita Karani

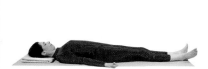

41 · Savasana

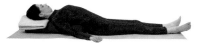

41 · Savasana (on bolsters)

POINTS TO PRACTISE

Standing Poses
● Stand evenly on the inner and outer edges of the feet, and on the heels and mounds of the toes.

● Stretch the toes.
● Tighten the knees and pull up the thigh muscles.
● Keep the back leg strong and stable while bending the front leg.
● Make a right angle accurately.

● In turned poses, turn the hips to the maximum.
● Open the palms and extend fingers.
● Turn the head and neck without straining.
● Keep the face relaxed.

WEEK 2

MONDAY, WEDNESDAY AND FRIDAY

1 · *Tadasana*
3 · *Trikonasana*
4 · *Parsvakonasana*
6 · *Virabhadrasana II*
*7 · *Parsvottanasana (simple)*
9 · *Uttanasana*
*31 · *Adho Mukha Svanasana*
16 · *Virasana (forward bend)*
34 · *Sarvangasana*
*35 · *Halasana*
41 · *Savasana*

TUESDAY AND THURSDAY

*33 · *Bharadvajasana (on chair)*
14 · *Sukhasana*
17 · *Parvatasana (in Sukhasana)*
*15 · *Virasana*
*17 · *Parvatasana (in Virasana)*
20 · *Gomukhasana (arms only)*
31 · *Adho Mukha Svanasana*
34 · *Sarvangasana*
35 · *Halasana*
41 · *Savasana*

SATURDAY

31 · *Adho Mukha Svanasana*
9 · *Uttanasana (on ledge)*
1 · *Tadasana*
2 · *Vrksasana*
3 · *Trikonasana*
4 · *Parsvakonasana*
6 · *Virabhadrasana II*
*7 · *Parsvottanasana (full pose)*
16 · *Virasana (forward bend)*
34 · *Sarvangasana*
35 · *Halasana*
41 · *Savasana*

SUNDAY

26 · *Cross Bolsters*
27 · *Matsyasana (simple)*
31 · *Adho Mukha Svanasana (head supported)*
9 · *Uttanasana*
39 · *Setu Bandha Sarvangasana (on bolster)*
40 · *Viparita Karani*
41 · *Savasana (on bolster)*

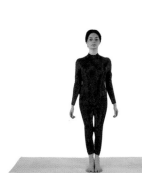

1 · Tadasana

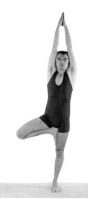

2 · Vrksasana

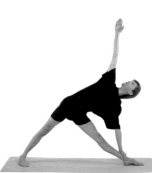

3 · Trikonasana

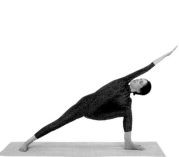

4 · Parsvakonasana

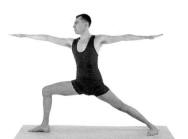

6 · Virabhadrasana II

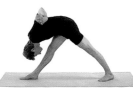

7 · Parsvottanasana (simple)

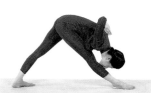

7 · Parsvottanasana (full pose)

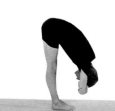

9 · Uttanasana

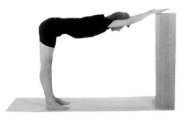

9 · *Uttanasana*
(on ledge)

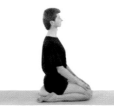

14 · *Sukhasana*

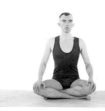

15 · *Virasana*

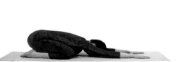

16 · *Virasana*
(forward bend)

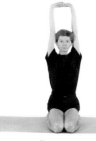

17 · *Parvatasana*
(in Virasana)

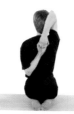

20 · *Gomukhasana*
(arms only)

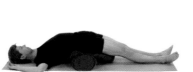

26 · *Cross Bolsters*

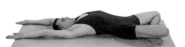

27 · *Matsyasana (simple)*

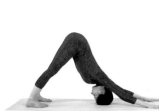

31 · *Adho Mukha*
Svanasana

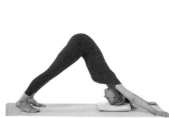

31 · *Adho Mukha*
Svanasana
(head supported)

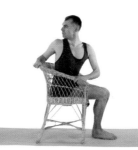

33 · *Bharadvajasana*
(on chair)

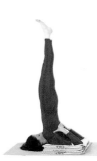

34 · *Sarvangasana*

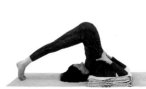

35 · *Halasana*

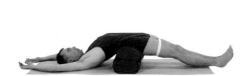

39 · *Setu Bandha*
Sarvangasana
(on bolster)

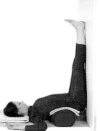

40 · *Viparita Karani*

41 · *Savasana*

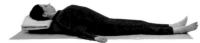

41 · *Savasana*
(on bolster)

WEEK 3

MONDAY, WEDNESDAY AND FRIDAY

- 31 · *Adho Mukha Svanasana*
- 9 · *Uttanasana (on ledge)*
- 1 · *Tadasana*
- 3 · *Trikonasana*
- 4 · *Parsvakonasana*
- 6 · *Virabhadrasana II*
- *5 · *Virabhadrasana I*
- 9 · *Uttanasana*
- *7 · *Parsvottanasana (full pose)*
- 33 · *Bharadvajasana (on a chair)*
- 14 · *Sukhasana*
- 17 · *Parvatasana (in Sukhasana)*
- 34 · *Sarvangasana*
- 35 · *Halasana*
- 41 · *Savasana*

TUESDAY AND THURSDAY

- 9 · *Uttanasana*
- 31 · *Adho Mukha Svanasana*
- *18 · *Dandasana*
- *22 · *Triang Mukhaikapada Pascimottanasana (concave)*
- *24 · *Pascimottanasana (concave)*
- 36 · *Ardha Halasana*
- *39 · *Setu Bandha Sarvangasana (on bolster)*
- *30 · *Urdhva Prasarita Padasana*
- 41 · *Savasana*

SATURDAY

- 33 · *Bharadvajasana (on a chair)*
- *32 · *Maricyasana (standing)*
- 1 · *Tadasana*
- 3 · *Trikonasana*
- 4 · *Parsvakonasana*
- 6 · *Virabhadrasana II*
- 5 · *Virabhadrasana I*
- 9 · *Uttanasana*
- 7 · *Parsvottanasana (full pose)*
- *11 · *Garudasana*
- 15 · *Virasana*
- 17 · *Parvatasana (in Virasana)*
- 16 · *Virasana (forward bend)*
- 34 · *Sarvangasana*
- 35 · *Halasana*
- 41 · *Savasana*

SUNDAY

- 26 · *Cross Bolsters*
- 27 · *Matsyasana (simple)*
- *28 · *Supta Baddhakonasana*
- 31 · *Adho Mukha Svanasana*
- 9 · *Uttanasana (on ledge)*
- *38 · *Sarvangasana (against wall)*
- 36 · *Ardha Halasana*
- 39 · *Setu Bandha Sarvangasana (on bolster)*
- 40 · *Viparita Karani*
- 41 · *Savasana (on bolster)*

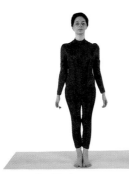

1 · Tadasana

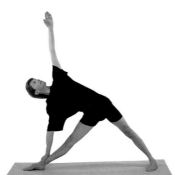

3 · Trikonasana

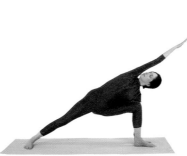

4 · Parsvakonasana

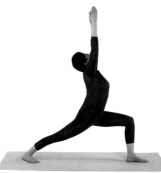

5 · Virabhadrasana I

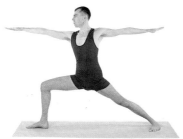

6 · Virabhadrasana II

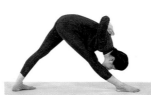

7 · Parsvottanasana (full pose)

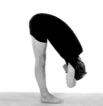

9 · Uttanasana

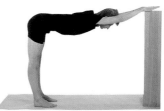

9 · Uttanasana (on ledge)

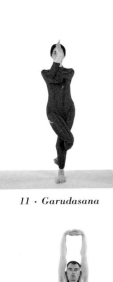

11 · Garudasana

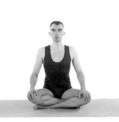

14 · Sukhasana

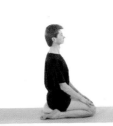

15 · Virasana

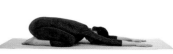

16 · Virasana
(forward bend)

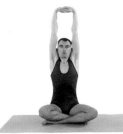

17 · Parvatasana
(in Sukhasana)

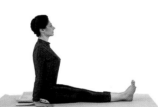

17 · Parvatasana
(in Virasana)

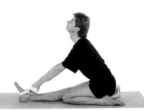

18 · Dandasana

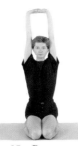

22 · Triang Mukhaikapada
Pascimottanasana
(concave)

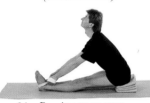

24 · Pascimottanasana
(concave)

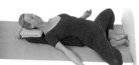

26 · Cross Bolsters

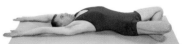

27 · Matsyasana

28 · Supta
Baddhakonasana

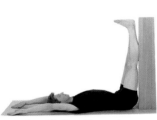

30 · Urdhva Prasarita
Padasana

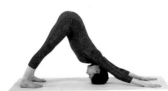

31 · Adho Mukha
Svanasana

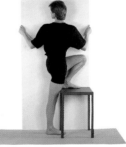

32 · Maricyasana
(standing)

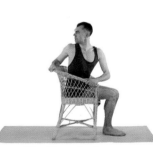

33 · Bharadvajasana
(on chair)

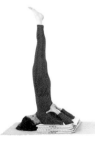

34 · Sarvangasana

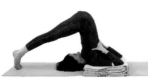

35 · Halasana

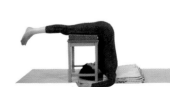

36 · Ardha Halasana

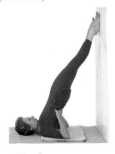

38 · Sarvangasana
(against wall)

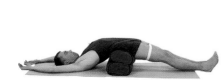

39 · Setu Bandha
Sarvangasana (on bolster)

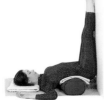

40 · Viparita Karani

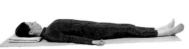

41 · Savasana

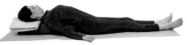

41 · Savasana
(on bolster)

WEEK 4

MONDAY, WEDNESDAY AND FRIDAY	TUESDAY AND THURSDAY	SATURDAY	SUNDAY
15 · *Virasana*	32 · *Maricyasana (standing)*	1 · *Tadasana*	26 · *Cross Bolsters*
*13 · *Utthita Hasta Padangusthasana (forward and sideways)*	33 · *Bharadvajasana (on chair)*	2 · *Vrksasana*	27 · *Matsyasana (simple)*
1 · *Tadasana*	31 · *Adho Mukha Svanasana*	3 · *Trikonasana*	28 · *Supta Baddhakonasana*
3 · *Trikonasana*	18 · *Dandasana*	4 · *Parsvakonasana*	31 · *Adho Mukha Svanasana*
4 · *Parsvakonasana*	*21 · *Janusirsasana (concave)*	6 · *Virabhadrasana II*	9 · *Uttanasana (on ledge)*
6 · *Virabhadrasana II*	22 · *Triang Mukhaikapada Pascimottanasana (concave)*	5 · *Virabhadrasana I*	38 · *Sarvangasana (against wall)*
5 · *Virabhadrasana I*	*23 · *Maricyasana I (twist only)*	9 · *Uttanasana*	36 · *Ardha Halasana*
9 · *Uttanasana*	24 · *Pascimottanasana (concave)*	7 · *Parsvottanasana (full pose)*	39 · *Setu Bandha Sarvangasana (on bolster)*
7 · *Parsvottanasana (full pose)*	*25 · *Malasana (preparatory)*	11 · *Garudasana*	40 · *Viparita Karani*
17 · *Virasana (forward bend)*	34 · *Sarvangasana*	20 · *Gomukhasana (arms only)*	41 · *Savasana (on bolster)*
14 · *Sukhasana*	35 · *Halasana*	31 · *Adho Mukha Svanasana*	
27 · *Matsyasana*	41 · *Savasana*	34 · *Sarvangasana*	
34 · *Sarvangasana*		36 · *Ardha Halasana*	
35 · *Halasana*		41 · *Savasana*	
41 · *Savasana*			

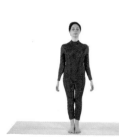 1 · *Tadasana*
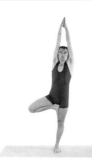 2 · *Vrksasana*
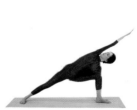 3 · *Trikonasana*
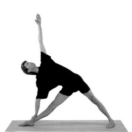 4 · *Parsvakonasana*
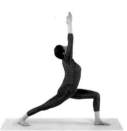 5 · *Virabhadrasana I*
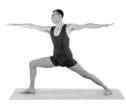 6 · *Virabhadrasana II*
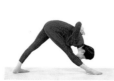 7 · *Parsvottanasana*
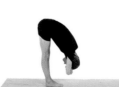 9 · *Uttanasana*
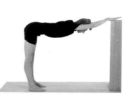 9 · *Uttanasana (on ledge)*
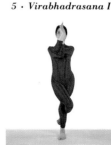 11 · *Garudasana*

Standing Poses
● Stretch legs up from ankle bones.
● In forward-facing poses, open the hips outward.
● Extend the front, sides and back of the body.

Sitting Poses
● Adjust the height of support in order not to slump in the lower back or push the lumber forward.
● In concave poses, lift and open the chest and move the back ribs in.

● In bent-legged poses, relax the groins and knees; take the thighs down without collapsing the back.
● In poses with straight legs, extend the legs and keep the thighs and knees down.

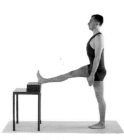

13 · Utthita Hasta Padangusthasana (forward)

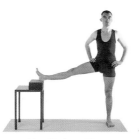

13 · Utthita Hasta Padangusthasana (sideways)

14 · Sukhasana

15 · Virasana

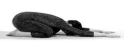

16 · Virasana (forward bend)

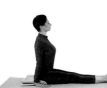

18 · Dandasana

20 · Gomukhasana

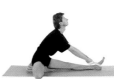

21 · Janusirsasana (concave)

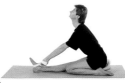

22 · Triang Mukhaikapada Pascimottanasana (concave)

23 · Maricyasana I

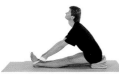

24 · Pascimottanasana (concave)

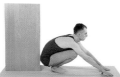

25 · Malasana (preparatory)

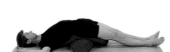

26 · Cross Bolsters

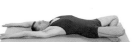

27 · Matsyasana

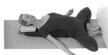

28 · Supta Baddhakonasana

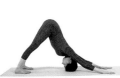

31 · Adho Mukha Svanasana

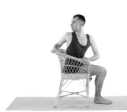

32 · Maricyasana (standing)

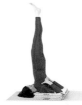

33 · Bharadvajasana (on chair)

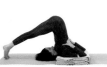

34 · Sarvangasana

35 · Halasana

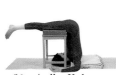

36 · Ardha Halasana

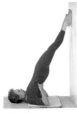

38 · Sarvangasana (against wall)

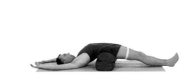

39 · Setu Bandha Sarvangasana (on bolster)

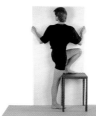

40 · Viparita Karani

41 · Savasana

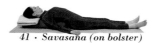

41 · Savasana (on bolster)

WEEK 5

Practise a mixture of dynamic and resting programmes from the previous four weeks.

WEEK 6

MONDAY, WEDNESDAY AND FRIDAY

1 · *Tadasana*
3 · *Trikonasana*
4 · *Parsvakonasana*
5 · *Virabhadrasana I*
9 · *Uttanasana*
6 · *Virabhadrasana II*
7 · *Parsvottanasana (full pose)*
*8 · *Prasarita Padottanasana*
16 · *Virasana (forward bend)*
34 · *Sarvangasana*
35 · *Halasana*
24 · *Pascimottanasana*
30 · *Urdhva Prasarita Padasana*
41 · *Savasana*

TUESDAY AND THURSDAY

9 · *Uttanasana*
31 · *Adho Mukha Svanasana*
*21 · *Janusirsasana (head supported)*
*22 · *Triang Mukhaikapada Pascimottanasana (head supported)*
*24 · *Pascimottanasana (head supported)*
23 · *Maricyasana I (twist only)*
34 · *Sarvangasana*
36 · *Ardha Halasana*
*39 · *Setu Bandha Sarvangasana (on bench)*
41 · *Savasana*

SATURDAY

13 · *Utthita Hasta Padangusthasana (forward and sideways)*
1 · *Tadasana*
3 · *Trikonasana*
4 · *Parsvakonasana*
5 · *Virabhadrasana I*
9 · *Uttanasana*
6 · *Virabhadrasana II*
7 · *Parsvottanasana (arms stretched)*
8 · *Prasarita Padottanasana*
*12 · *Utkatasana*
25 · *Malasana (preparatory)*
16 · *Virasana (forward bend)*
36 · *Ardha Halasana*
34 · *Sarvangasana*
41 · *Savasana*

SUNDAY

31 · *Adho Mukha Svanasana (head supported)*
16 · *Virasana (forward bend)*
9 · *Uttanasana*
30 · *Urdhva Prasarita Padasana*
27 · *Matsyasana (simple)*
28 · *Supta Baddhakonasana*
*37 · *Sarvangasana (on chair)*
36 · *Ardha Halasana*
41 · *Savasana (on bolster) (1) relaxing (2) observing the breath*

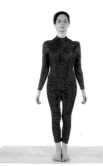

1 · *Tadasana*

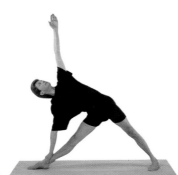

3 · *Trikonasana*

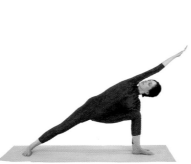

4 · *Parsvakonasana*

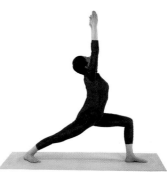

5 · *Virabhadrasana I*

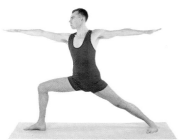

6 · *Virabhadrasana II*

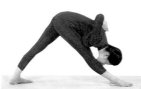

7 · *Parsvottanasana (full pose)*

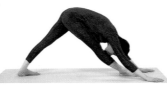

7 · *Parsvottanasana (arms stretched)*

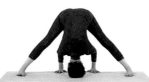

8 · *Prasarita Padottanasana*

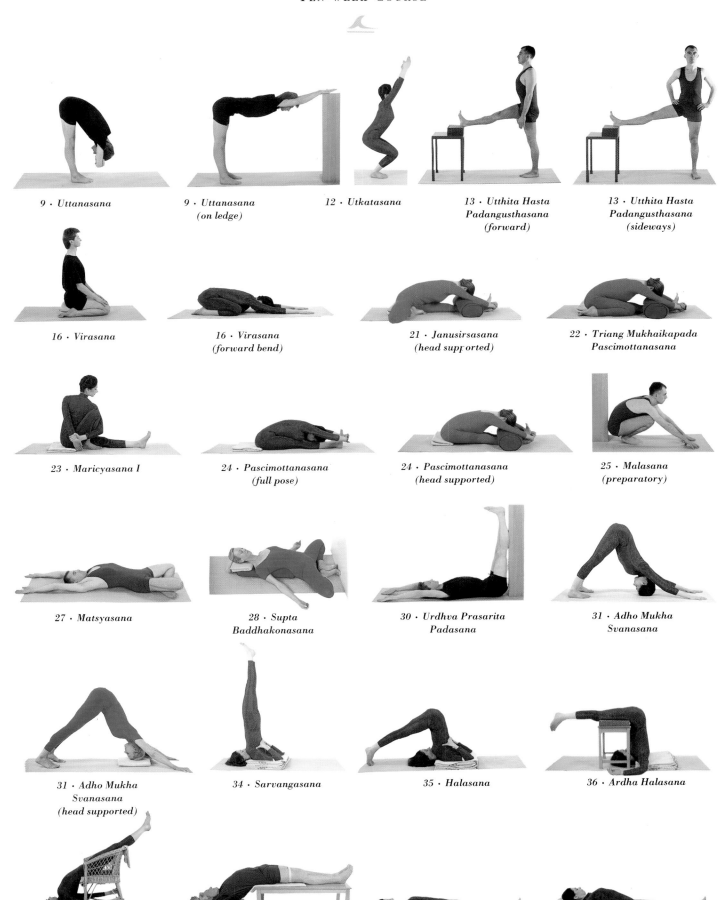

9 · *Uttanasana*

9 · *Uttanasana*
(on ledge)

12 · *Utkatasana*

13 · *Utthita Hasta*
Padangusthasana
(forward)

13 · *Utthita Hasta*
Padangusthasana
(sideways)

16 · *Virasana*

16 · *Virasana*
(forward bend)

21 · *Janusirsasana*
(head supported)

22 · *Triang Mukhaikapada*
Pascimottanasana

23 · *Maricyasana I*

24 · *Pascimottanasana*
(full pose)

24 · *Pascimottanasana*
(head supported)

25 · *Malasana*
(preparatory)

27 · *Matsyasana*

28 · *Supta*
Baddhakonasana

30 · *Urdhva Prasarita*
Padasana

31 · *Adho Mukha*
Svanasana

31 · *Adho Mukha*
Svanasana
(head supported)

34 · *Sarvangasana*

35 · *Halasana*

36 · *Ardha Halasana*

37 · *Sarvangasana*
(on chair)

39 · *Setu Bandha*
Sarvangasana (on bench)

41 · *Savasana*

41 · *Savasana*
(on bolster)

WEEK 7

MONDAY, WEDNESDAY AND FRIDAY

- 15 · *Virasana*
- 31 · *Adho Mukha Svanasana*
- 1 · *Tadasana*
- 3 · *Trikonasana*
- 4 · *Parsvakonasana*
- 5 · *Virabhadrasana I*
- 9 · *Uttanasana*
- 6 · *Virabhadrasana II*
- 7 · *Parsvottanasana*
- 8 · *Prasarita Padottanasana*
- 16 · *Virasana (forward bend)*
- *29 · *Supta Virasana*
- 28 · *Supta Baddhakonasana*
- 34 · *Sarvangasana*
- 35 · *Halasana*
- 24 · *Pascimottanasana*
- 41 · *Savasana*

TUESDAY AND THURSDAY

- 32 · *Maricyasana (standing)*
- 33 · *Bharadvajasana (on chair)*
- 9 · *Uttanasana (on ledge)*
- 31 · *Adho Mukha Svanasana*
- 14 · *Sukhasana*
- 17 · *Parvatasana (in Sukhasana)*
- 15 · *Virasana*
- 17 · *Parvatasana (in Virasana)*
- 18 · *Dandasana*
- *19 · *Siddhasana*
- 20 · *Gomukhasana (arms only)*
- * *Namaste (in Virasana)*
- 34 · *Sarvangasana*
- 35 · *Halasana*
- 41 · *Savasana*

SATURDAY

- 14 · *Sukhasana*
- 15 · *Virasana*
- 17 · *Parvatasana (in Virasana)*
- 31 · *Adho Mukha Svanasana*
- 18 · *Dandasana*
- 21 · *Janusirsasana (concave)*
- 22 · *Triang Mukhaikapada Pascimottanasana (concave)*
- 24 · *Pascimottanasana (concave)*
- 23 · *Maricyasana I (twist only)*
- *33 · *Bharadvajasana (preparatory)*
- 25 · *Malasana (preparatory)*
- 34 · *Sarvangasana*
- 35 · *Halasana*
- 41 · *Savasana*

SUNDAY

- 31 · *Adho Mukha Svanasana (head supported)*
- 16 · *Virasana (forward bend)*
- 9 · *Uttanasana*
- 30 · *Urdhva Prasarita Padasana*
- 27 · *Matsyasana (simple)*
- 28 · *Supta Baddhakonasana*
- 37 · *Sarvangasana (on chair)*
- 36 · *Ardha Halasana*
- 41 · *Savasana (on bolster) (1) relaxing (2) observing the breath*

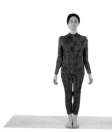

1 · *Tadasana*

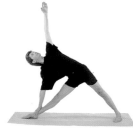

3 · *Trikonasana*

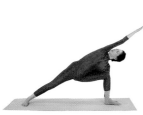

4 · *Parsvakonasana*

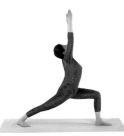

5 · *Virabhadrasana I*

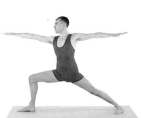

6 · *Virabhadrasana II*

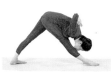

7 · *Parsvottanasana*

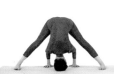

8 · *Prasarita Padottanasana*

9 · *Uttanasana*

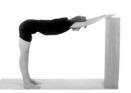

9 · *Uttanasana (on ledge)*

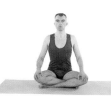

14 · *Sukhasana*

Sitting Poses

● In forward-bending poses, lengthen the whole trunk.
● Look up without compressing the back of the neck.

● Extend the upper arms away from the shoulders, the forearms away from the elbows, and the hands away from the wrists.
● Catch further and further.

Twists

● Keep the legs stable as you turn.
● Move the whole trunk when turning. ● Catch further. ● Turn the head without tensing the neck.

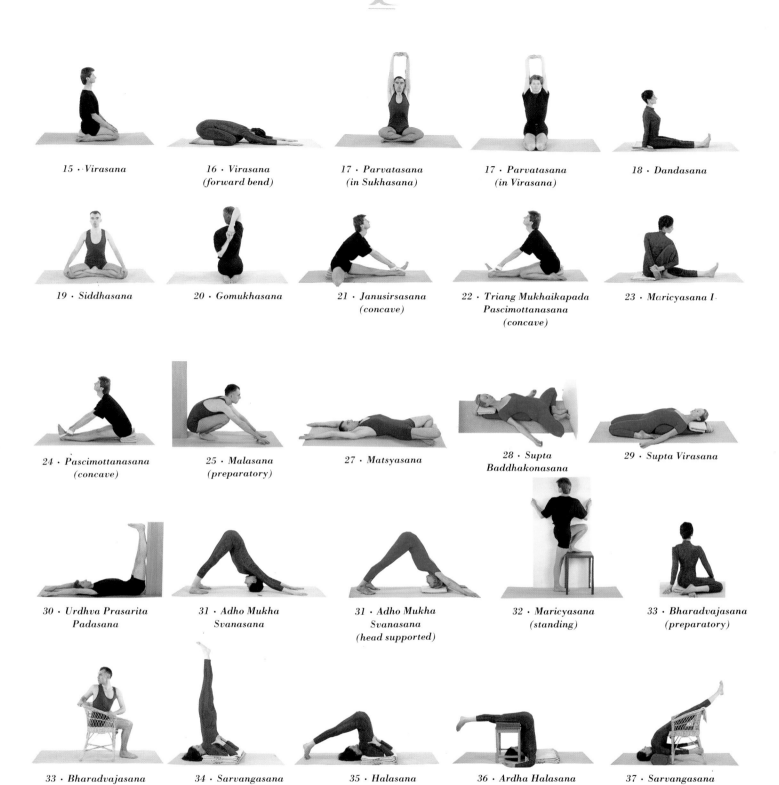

15 · *Virasana*

16 · *Virasana*
(forward bend)

17 · *Parvatasana*
(in Sukhasana)

17 · *Parvatasana*
(in Virasana)

18 · *Dandasana*

19 · *Siddhasana*

20 · *Gomukhasana*

21 · *Janusirsasana*
(concave)

22 · *Triang Mukhaikapada*
Pascimottanasana
(concave)

23 · *Maricyasana I*

24 · *Pascimottanasana*
(concave)

25 · *Malasana*
(preparatory)

27 · *Matsyasana*

28 · *Supta*
Baddhakonasana

29 · *Supta Virasana*

30 · *Urdhva Prasarita*
Padasana

31 · *Adho Mukha*
Svanasana

31 · *Adho Mukha*
Svanasana
(head supported)

32 · *Maricyasana*
(standing)

33 · *Bharadvajasana*
(preparatory)

33 · *Bharadvajasana*
(on chair)

34 · *Sarvangasana*

35 · *Halasana*

36 · *Ardha Halasana*

37 · *Sarvangasana*
(on chair)

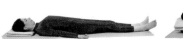

41 · *Savasana*

41 · *Savasana*
(on boster)

WEEK 8

MONDAY, WEDNESDAY AND FRIDAY

1 · *Tadasana*
2 · *Vrksasana*
3 · *Trikonasana*
4 · *Parsvakonasana*
5 · *Virabhadrasana I*
9 · *Uttanasana*
6 · *Virabhadrasana II*
7 · *Parsvottanasana (full pose)*
9 · *Uttanasana*
*10 · *Padangusthasana*
12 · *Utkatasana*
11 · *Garudasana*
16 · *Virasana (forward bend)*
36 · *Ardha Halasana*
41 · *Savasana*

TUESDAY AND THURSDAY

9 · *Uttanasana (on ledge)*
31 · *Adho Mukha Svanasana*
16 · *Virasana (forward bend)*
18 · *Dandasana*
*21 · *Janusirsasana (full pose)*
*22 · *Triang Mukhaikapada Pascimottanasana (full pose)*
*24 · *Pascimottanasana (full pose)*
33 · *Bharadvajasana (preparatory)*
36 · *Ardha Halasana*
39 · *Setu Bandha Sarvangasana (on bench)*
40 · *Viparita Karani*
41 · *Savasana*

SATURDAY

33 · *Bharadvajasana (on chair)*
32 · *Maricyasana (standing)*
1 · *Tadasana*
3 · *Trikonasana*
4 · *Parsvakonasana*
5 · *Virabhadrasana I*
9 · *Uttanasana*
6 · *Virabhadrasana II*
7 · *Parsvottanasana (arms stretched)*
8 · *Prasarita Padottanasana*
25 · *Malasana (preparatory)*
31 · *Adho Mukha Svanasana*
16 · *Virasana (forward bend)*
34 · *Sarvangasana*
35 · *Halasana*
41 · *Savasana*

SUNDAY

26 · *Cross Bolsters*
27 · *Matsyasana*
28 · *Supta Baddhakonasana*
29 · *Supta Virasana*
16 · *Virasana (forward bend)*
9 · *Uttanasana*
31 · *Adho Mukha Svanasana*
37 · *Sarvangasana (on chair)*
36 · *Ardha Halasana*
39 · *Setu Bandha Sarvangasana (on bench)*
41 · *Savasana (on bolster)*
  (1) *relaxing*
  (2) *observing the breath*
  (3) *lengthening the breath*

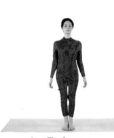

1 · Tadasana

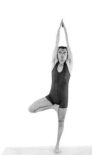

2 · Vrksasana

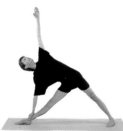

3 · Trikonasana

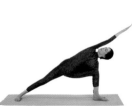

4 · Parsvakonasana

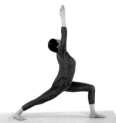

5 · Virabhadrasana I

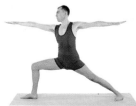

6 · Virabhadrasana II

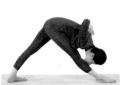

7 · Parsvottanasana

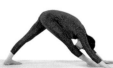

7 · Parsvottanasana (arms stretched)

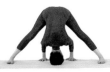

8 · Prasarita Padottanasana

9 · Uttanasana

Prone and Supine Poses
● Extend the front of the body and keep it relaxed; enjoy opening the chest; breathe evenly.

● In supported poses find the best position.
● Place the head and neck in a comfortable position.

Inverted Poses
● In supported poses, experiment with the height of the support to make it most effective.

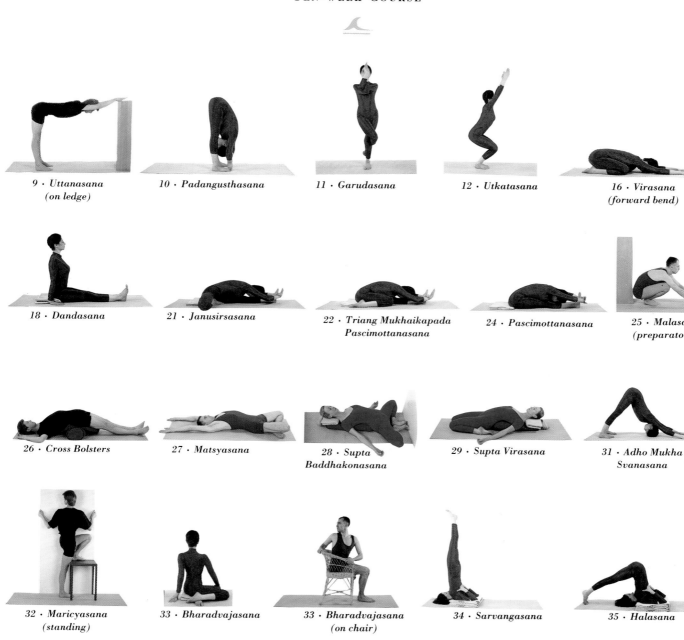

9 · *Uttanasana*
(on ledge)

10 · *Padangusthasana*

11 · *Garudasana*

12 · *Utkatasana*

16 · *Virasana*
(forward bend)

18 · *Dandasana*

21 · *Janusirsasana*

22 · *Triang Mukhaikapada Pascimottanasana*

24 · *Pascimottanasana*

25 · *Malasana*
(preparatory)

26 · *Cross Bolsters*

27 · *Matsyasana*

28 · *Supta Baddhakonasana*

29 · *Supta Virasana*

31 · *Adho Mukha Svanasana*

32 · *Maricyasana*
(standing)

33 · *Bharadvajasana*

33 · *Bharadvajasana*
(on chair)

34 · *Sarvangasana*

35 · *Halasana*

36 · *Ardha Halasana*

37 · *Sarvangasana*
(on chair)

39 · *Setu Bandha Sarvangasana*
(on bench)

40 · *Viparita Karani*

41 · *Savasana*

41 · *Savasana*
(on bolster)

● Keep the chest open and lifted while remaining relaxed.
● Keep the head in line with the rest of the body.

● Extend the neck without tension.
● Adjust the arms and shoulders to make them even, and get in a comfortable position.

Relaxation
● Place yourself accurately.
● Breathe quietly.
● Relax, letting go completely.

WEEK 9

MONDAY, WEDNESDAY AND FRIDAY	TUESDAY AND THURSDAY	SATURDAY	SUNDAY
13 · *Utthita Hasta Padangusthasana (forward and sideways)*	15 · *Virasana*	1 · *Tadasana*	26 · *Cross Bolsters*
1 · *Tadasana*	17 · *Parvatasana (in Virasana)*	2 · *Vrksasana*	27 · *Matsyasana*
3 · *Trikonasana*	14 · *Sukhasana*	11 · *Garudasana*	28 · *Supta Baddhakonasana*
4 · *Parsvakonasana*	17 · *Parvatasana (in Sukhasana)*	12 · *Utkatasana*	29 · *Supta Virasana*
5 · *Virabhadrasana I*	20 · *Gomukhasana (arms only)*	15 · *Virasana*	16 · *Virasana (forward bend)*
9 · *Uttanasana*	33 · *Bharadvajasana (on chair)*	19 · *Siddhasana*	9 · *Uttanasana*
6 · *Virabhadrasana II*	32 · *Maricyasana (standing)*	18 · *Dandasana*	31 · *Adho Mukha Svanasana*
7 · *Parsvottanasana*	18 · *Dandasana*	21 · *Janusirsasana*	37 · *Sarvangasana (on chair)*
8 · *Prasarita Padottanasana*	23 · *Maricyasana I (twist only)*	22 · *Triang Mukhaikapada Pascimottanasana*	36 · *Ardha Halasana*
10 · *Padangusthasana*	*33 · *Bharadvajasana*	24 · *Pascimottanasana*	39 · *Setu Bandha Sarvangasana (on bench)*
31 · *Adho Mukha Svanasana*	25 · *Malasana*	31 · *Adho Mukha Svanasana*	41 · *Savasana (on bolster) (1) relaxing (2) observing the breath (3) lengthening the breath*
16 · *Virasana (forward bend)*	34 · *Sarvangasana*	34 · *Sarvangasana*	
34 · *Sarvangasana*	35 · *Halasana*	35 · *Halasana*	
21 · *Janusirsasana*	24 · *Pascimottanasana*	41 · *Savasana*	
24 · *Pascimottanasana*	41 · *Savasana*		
41 · *Savasana*			

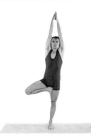
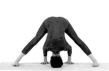

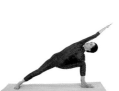
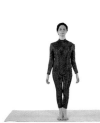

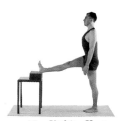
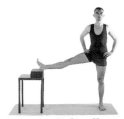
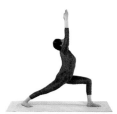
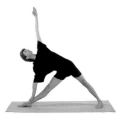

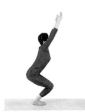
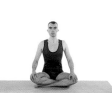
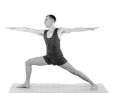
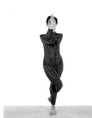

1 · Tadasana

2 · Vrksasana

3 · Trikonasana

4 · Parsvakonasana

5 · Virabhadrasana I

6 · Virabhadrasana II

7 · Parsvottanasana

8 · Prasarita Padottanasana

9 · Uttanasana

10 · Padangusthasana

11 · Garudasana

12 · Utkatasana

13 · Utthita Hasta Padangusthasana (forward)

13 · Utthita Hasta Padangusthasana (sideways)

14 · Sukhasana

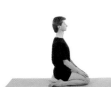

15 · *Virasana*

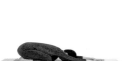

16 · *Virasana*
(forward bend)

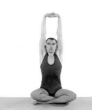
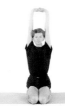

17 · *Parvatasana*
(in Sukhasana)

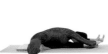

17 · *Parvatasana*
(in Virasana)

18 · *Dandasana*

19 · *Siddhasana*

20 · *Gomukhasana*
(arms only)

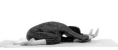

21 · *Janusirsasana*

22 · *Triang Mukhaikapada*
Pascimottanasana

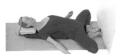

23 · *Maricyasana I*

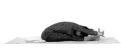

24 · *Pascimottanasana*

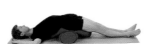

25 · *Malasana*
(preparatory)

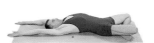

26 · *Cross Bolsters*

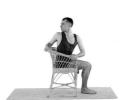

27 · *Matsyasana*

28 · *Supta*
Baddhakonasana

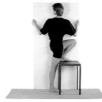

29 · *Supta*
Virasana

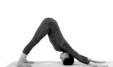

31 · *Adho Mukha*
Svanasana

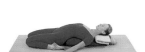

32 · *Maricyasana*
(standing)

33 · *Bharadvajasana*

33 · *Bharadvajasana*
(on chair)

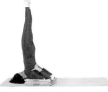

34 · *Sarvangasana*

35 · *Halasana*

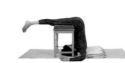

36 · *Ardha Halasana*

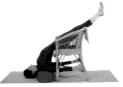

37 · *Sarvangasana*
(on chair)

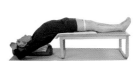

39 · *Setu Bandha*
Sarvangasana

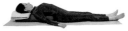

41 · *Savasana*

41 · *Savasana (on bolster)*

WEEK 10

Practise any programmes from weeks 6-9 inclusive.

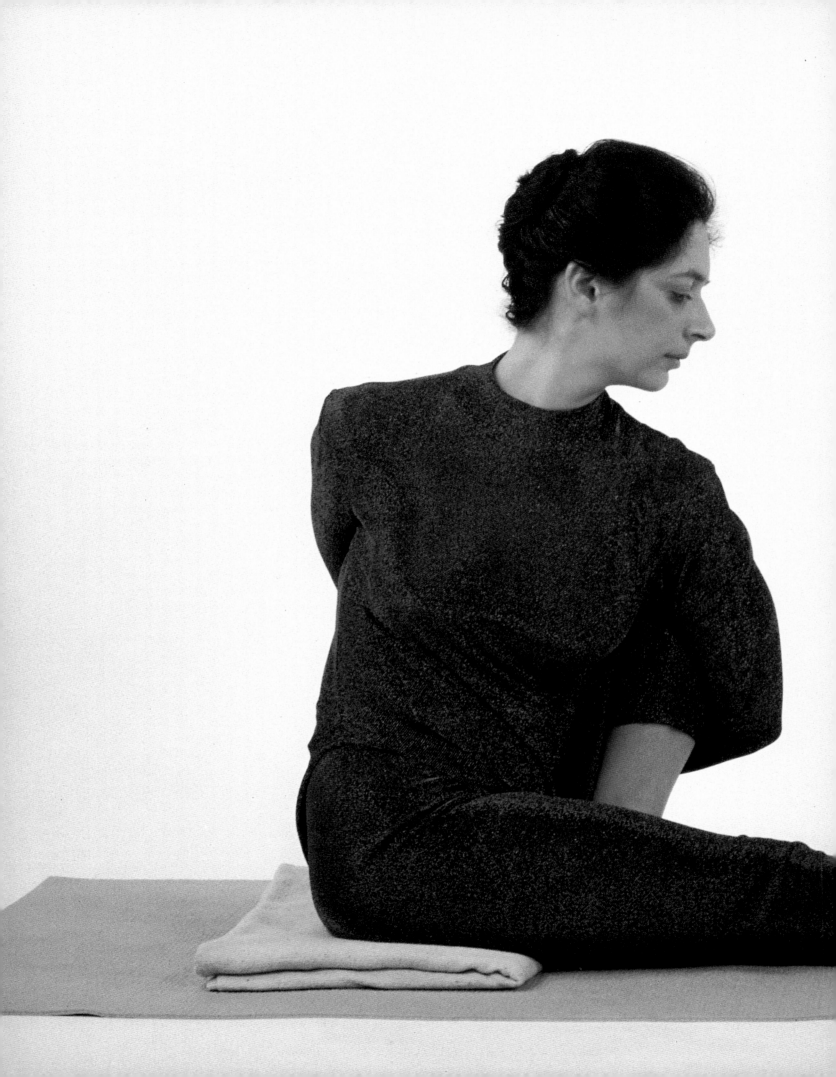

ASANAS FOR COMMON PROBLEMS

Although yoga should not be practised without advice if you suffer from serious ailments (see page 11) special postures have been recommended to offer relief from common problems such as headaches, stiffness in parts of the body and backache. If you have difficulty with any of these programmes then consult an experienced teacher.

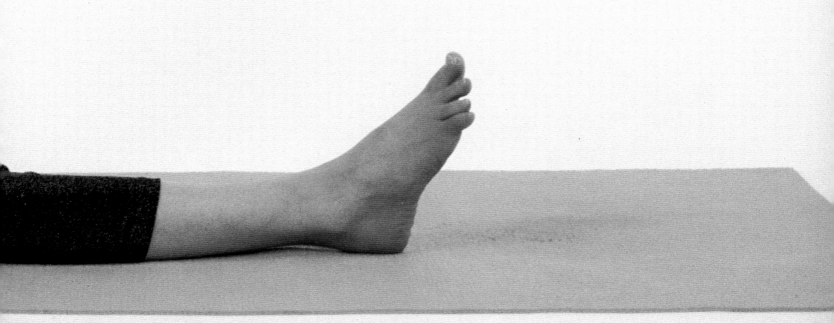

ASANAS FOR MENSTRUATION

Although menstruation is a normal and natural process, it involves physiological and metabolic changes, and yoga practice takes account of the altered condition of the body at this time. The postures given in this programme are a combination of restful ones and those that ease pain and strain.

Strenuous postures such as standing and inverted poses, and vigorous extensions in any poses, should be avoided. Yoga practice generally helps complaints associated with the menstrual cycle, such as cramp, irregularity, scanty or excessive bleeding, backache and pre-menstrual tension.

SUPTA VIRASANA
HERO POSE (SUPINE)

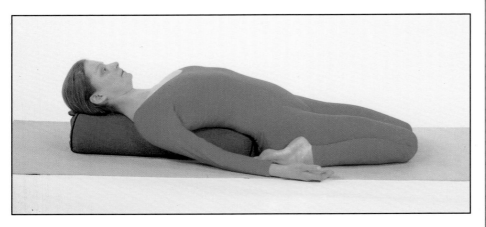

Do Supta Virasana (no. 29). Stay for 3–5 minutes, then come up.

SUPTA BADDHAKONASANA
SUPINE COBBLER POSE

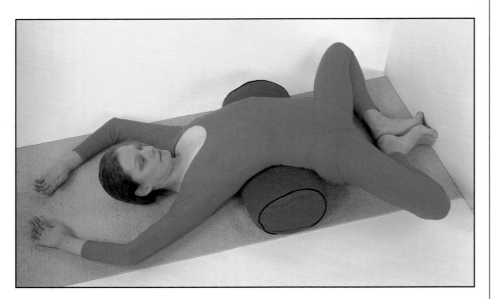

Do Supta Baddhakonasana (no. 28) with a crosswise bolster under *the waist. Stay for 5–8 minutes, then come up.*

BADDHAKONASANA
COBBLER POSE

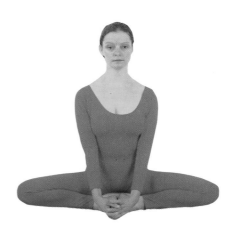

Sit in Dandasana (no. 18) against a wall, on one or two folded blankets. Bend the knees to the sides. Bring the feet together and line them up, with the soles touching. Bring the heels as close as possible to the pubis. Hold the toes. If you are sitting too high to reach them, hold the ankles. Stretch the thighs toward the knees and take the knees down. Stretch the trunk up and open the chest. Keep the head level.

Stay for 3–5 minutes, then release.

UPAVISTAKONASANA
— WIDE-ANGLED SEATED POSE —

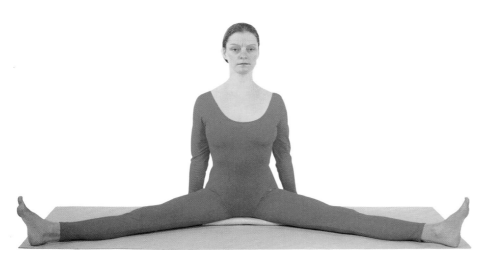

Sit in Dandasana (no. 18) on one or two folded blankets, with the back against a wall. Spread the legs apart, as wide as possible. Keep the front of the legs facing the ceiling and the feet upright. Straighten the knees and pull the thigh muscles back towards the groin. Draw the trunk up, extend the spine up and open the chest. Breathe evenly. Stay for 2–3 minutes, then release.

JANUSIRSASANA
— HEAD TO KNEE POSE —

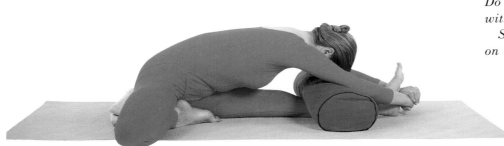

Do Janusirsasana (no. 21), variant with head supported.
Stay for 1–2 minutes, then repeat on the other side.

TRIANG MUKHAIKAPADA PASCIMOTTANASANA
— FORWARD BEND WITH LEG BENT BACK —

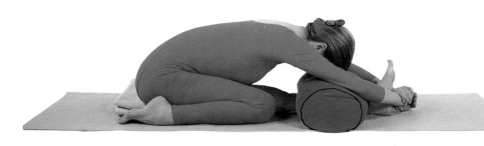

Do Triang Mukhaikapada Pascimottanasana (no. 22).
Stay for 1–2 minutes, then repeat on the other side.

- *If you experience cramp during menstruation, do the forward bends with the back concave.*
- *If you are stiff, rest the head on a stool.*
- *If there is strain in the knees, support it and reduce the length of time in the posture.*

ARDHA BADDHA PADMA PASCIMOTTANASANA
HALF-LOTUS FORWARD BEND

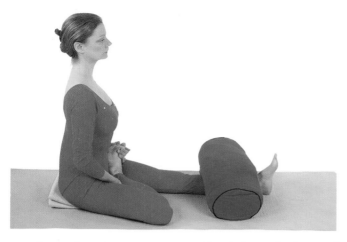

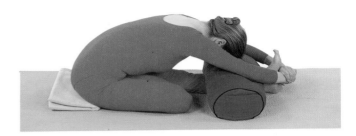

1 *Sit in Dandasana (no. 18). Bend the right leg and place the foot on top of the left thigh, in the groin. Place a bolster on the left shin.*

2 *Bend forward, hold the left foot and rest the head on the bolster. Stay for 30–40 seconds, then repeat on the other side.*

● *If there is strain in the knee, support it on a rolled blanket. Do not tense the knee.*

MARICYASANA I
SIMPLE TWIST WITH FORWARD BEND

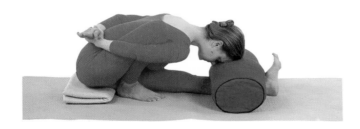

Do Maricyasana I (no. 23). Turn the trunk forward and bend down over the straight leg. Rest the head on the bolster. Keep the abdomen soft. Stay for 30–40 seconds, then repeat on the other side.

PASCIMOTTANASANA
FULL FORWARD BEND WITH HEAD SUPPORTED

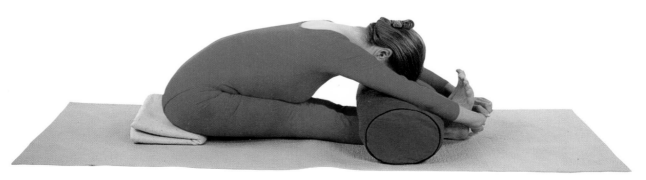

Do Pascimottanasana (no. 24) resting the head on a bolster. Stay for 2–3 minutes, then come up.

SETU BANDHA SARVANGASANA
NECK BALANCE BACK ARCH

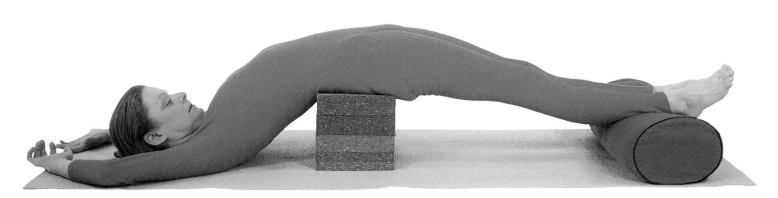

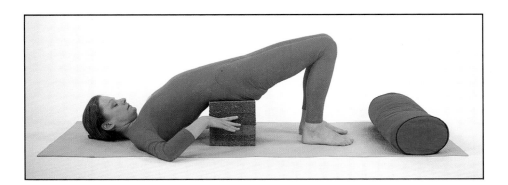

1 *Above: Do Setu Bandha Sarvangasana (no. 39). Lie over a support, such as a bench, folded blankets or bolsters. Stay for 5–8 minutes.*

2 *Left: To come down, bend the knees and hold the bench, blankets or bolsters. Slide back, then turn to the side and get up.*

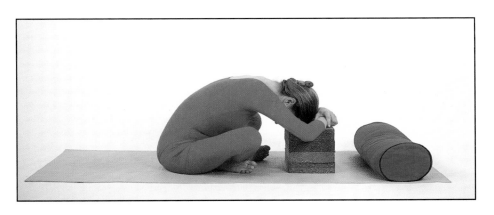

3 *Sit and bend forward, resting your head on the support. If the lower back pulls, take the buttocks a little further back, or sit on a bolster and bend down.*

SAVASANA
CORPSE POSE

Do Savasana (no. 41) for 5–10 minutes, then turn to the side and come up.

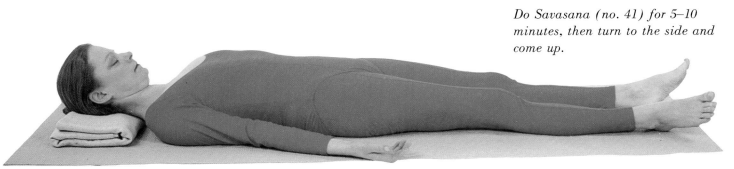

ASANAS FOR HEADACHES

The sequence of postures given here is designed to alleviate headaches caused by stress and tension.

The bandage, which we show wound round the head for the forward bends, can be used from the beginning. It relieves the internal pressure that comes with headaches. Care should be taken not to tie a bandage too tightly.

As you become stronger through regular yoga practice, you should find that you suffer less from headaches, and can get rid of them more easily.

CROSS BOLSTERS

Lie over Cross Bolsters (no. 26).

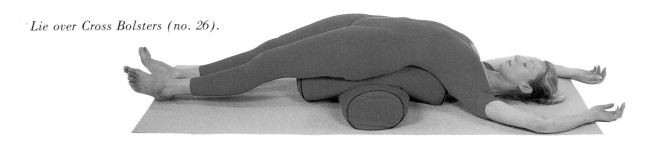

SUPTA VIRASANA
RECLINING HERO POSE

Do Supta Virasana (no. 29).

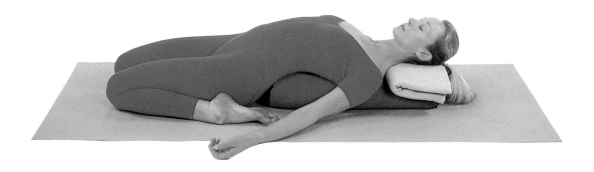

SUPTA BADDHAKONASANA
SUPINE COBBLER POSE

Do Supta Baddhakonasana (no. 28).

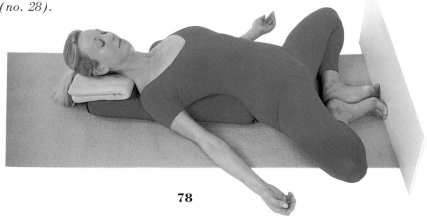

USING A BANDAGE

A firmly tied bandage round the head is very soothing for headaches. It cools the eyes, temples and head.

Wind a bandage several times round the forehead and back of the skull. Pull the bandage firmly but do not make it too tight.

If you have eyestrain also cover the eyes: in this case wind the bandage lightly two or three times round the eyes at the beginning.

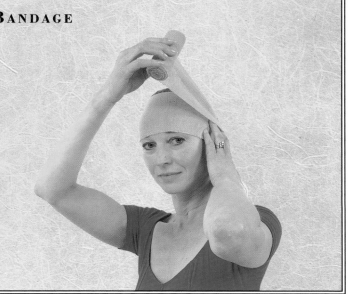

UTTANASANA
— STANDING BEND (HEAD SUPPORTED) —

Do Uttanasana (no. 9) as follows: place a folded blanket on a stool. Stand with the feet 12–18 inches (30–45 cm) apart in front of the stool. Bend down and rest the head on it. Fold the arms and relax.
Stay for 1–2 minutes, then come up.

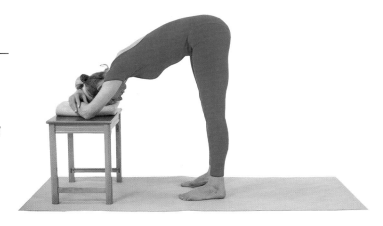

ADHO MUKHA SVANASANA
— DOG POSE (HEAD SUPPORTED) —

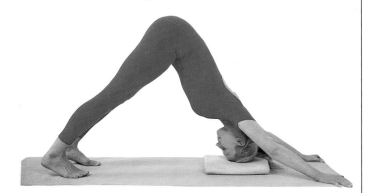

Do Adho Mukha Svanasana (no. 31), variant with head supported.

JANUSIRSASANA
HEAD-TO-KNEE POSE (HEAD SUPPORTED)

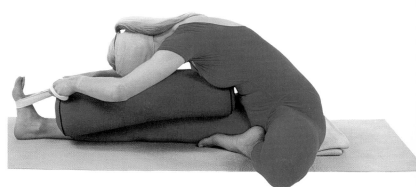

Do Janusirsasana (no. 21), variant with head on bolster, with the head bandaged. Place a bolster lengthwise on the extended leg and rest the head on it. If it is difficult to hold the foot, use a belt. Relax.
Stay for 2–5 minutes, then repeat on the other side.

PASCIMOTTANASANA
FULL FORWARD BEND (HEAD SUPPORTED)

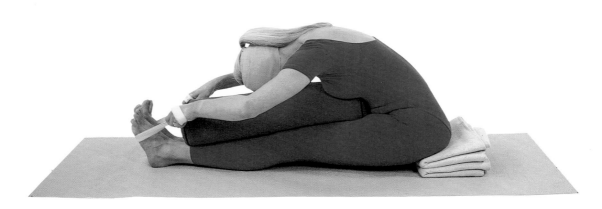

Do Pascimottanasana (no. 24) with the head bandaged. Place a bolster lengthwise on the legs and rest the head on it. Hold the feet with the hands or with a belt. Relax. Stay for 3–5 minutes,

ARDHA HALASANA
HALF-PLOUGH POSE

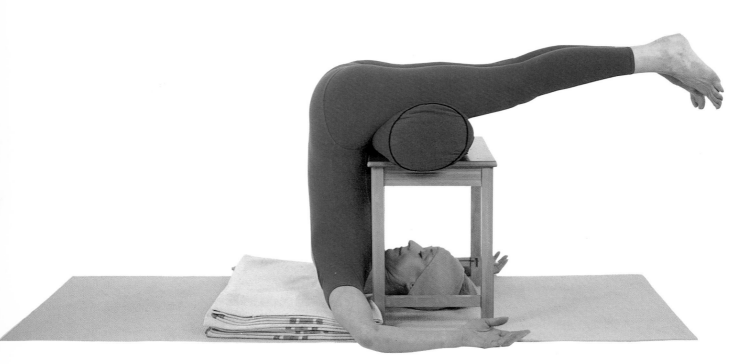

Do Ardha Halasana (no. 36). Stay for 5–8 minutes. To come down, bring the legs back a little, push the stool away and carefully slide down.

SETU BANDHA SARVANGASANA
NECK BALANCE WITH BACK ARCH

*Do Setu Bandha Sarvangasana
(no. 39), using two bolsters or a
pile of blankets under the lower
back. Support the legs if necessary.
Relax.*

*Stay for 5–8 minutes, then come
down.*

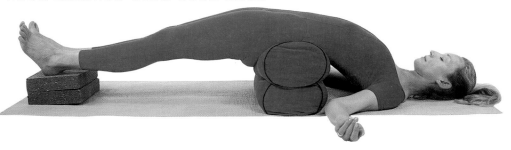

VIPARITA KARANI
RESTFUL INVERSION

*Do Viparita Karani (no. 40). Stay
for 5–8 minutes. Bend the knees,
slide backward, turn to the side
and get up.*

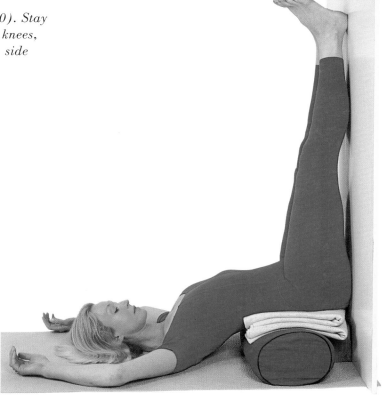

SAVASANA
CORPSE POSE

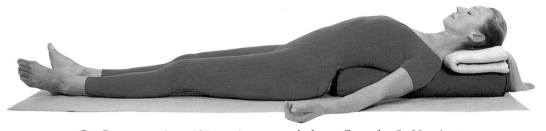

Do Savasana (no. 41), variant on a bolster. Stay for 5–10 minutes.

ASANAS FOR STIFF NECK AND SHOULDERS

The postures given here are designed to relieve stiffness and pain in the neck and shoulders. These problems are extremely common as well as troublesome; they are often caused by poor posture or life-style stress.

The postures emphasize freeing and stretching the affected areas to increase mobility. With time and regular practice, the neck and shoulders will become stronger and more supple, and will move to a more anatomically correct position. Gradually, pain and discomfort should diminish.

All the postures can be attempted by beginners.

TRIKONASANA
—— TRIANGLE POSE ——

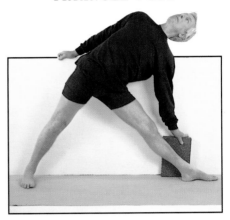

Do Trikonasana (no. 3) standing against a ledge or wall. Place one hand on a block and grip the ledge with the other hand to turn the trunk more. Stay for 20–30 seconds, then repeat on the other side.

PARSVAKONASANA
—— LATERAL ANGLE POSE ——

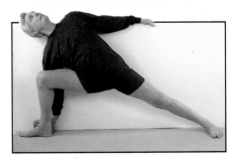

Do Parsvakonasana (no. 4), standing against a ledge or wall. Place the right hand on a block and grip the ledge with the left hand. Turn the trunk with the help of the hands. Stay for 20–30 seconds, then repeat on the other side.

ARDHA CANDRASANA
—— HALF-MOON POSE ——

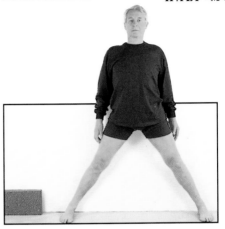

1 *Stand with your back 3–6 inches (7.5–15 cm) away from a ledge or wall. Take the feet 3½– 4 ft (105–120 cm) apart. Place a block against the wall, about 12 inches (30 cm) from the right foot.*

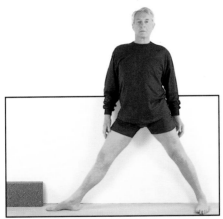

2 *Turn the left foot 15° in and the right foot 90° out.*

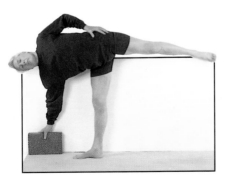

4 *Bring your weight onto the right foot and hand. At the same time, straighten the right leg and place the left foot on the ledge. Tighten both knees. Place the left hand on the left hip and turn the trunk forward. Keep the back against the wall. Stay for 20–30 seconds.*

To come down, bend the right leg and lower the left leg to the floor. Repeat on the other side.

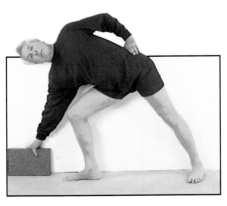

3 *Bend the right knee, lean sideways to the right and place the right hand on the block. Bring the left foot slightly in, toward the right foot. Hold the ledge.*

VIRASANA FORWARD BEND
——— HERO POSE ———

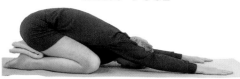

Do Virasana Forward Bend (no. 16). Place a bolster or folded blankets on the heels.

UTTANASANA WITH A POLE
STANDING FORWARD BEND

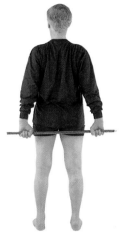

1 Stand with the feet hip-width apart. Hold a pole or stick horizontally behind the back, with the palms facing up.

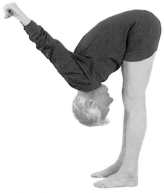

2 Bend forward and raise the pole up and over, as far as you can. Keep the elbows straight. Do not bend the knees. Stay for 10–20 seconds, then come up.

URDHVA MUKHA SVANASANA
——— DOG POSE HEAD UP (ON CHAIR) ———

Place a sturdy stool or chair against a wall. Grip the edges firmly with the hands. Bend the legs and rest the tops of the thighs on the seat. Step back and straighten the legs. Keep the arms firm, roll the shoulders back and stretch the trunk up. Curve the back and look up. Do not hold the breath. Stay for 15–20 seconds, then come down.

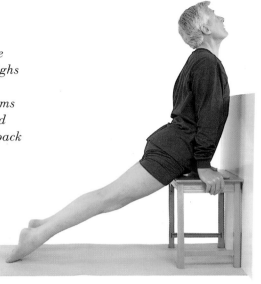

ADHO MUKHA SVANASANA
——— DOG POSE HEAD DOWN ———

Do Adho Mukha Svanasana (no. 31). Stretch the arms up strongly and lift the shoulders and trunk. Stay for 20–30 seconds, then come down.

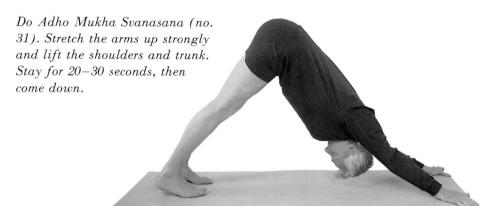

PARVATASANA IN VIRASANA
——— MOUNTAIN POSE ———

Do Parvatasana (no. 17), sitting in Virasana (no. 15). Stay for 20–30 seconds, then change the interlock of the fingers.

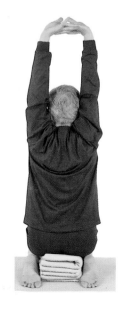

GOMUKHASANA (ARMS ONLY)
─── HEAD OF COW POSE ───

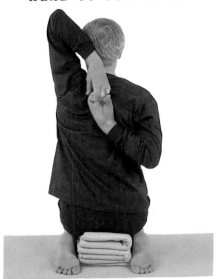

Sit in Virasana (no. 15). Catch the hands in Gomukhasana (no. 20). Stay for 20–30 seconds, then repeat on the other side.

NAMASTE (IN VIRASANA)
─── PRAYER POSITION ───

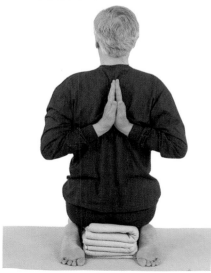

Sit in Virasana (no. 15) and join the palms behind the back in Namaste (no. 7). Stay for 30–60 seconds, then release. If the wrists hurt do not shake them but allow them to come to normal slowly.

BHARADVAJASANA
─── SIMPLE TWIST ───

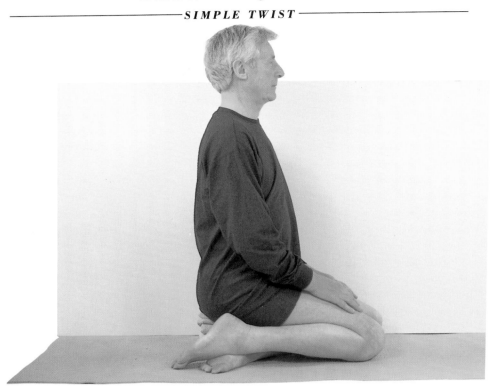

1 *Do Bharadvajasana (no. 33) sitting on one or two folded* | *blankets near a wall or ledge. Line yourself up.*

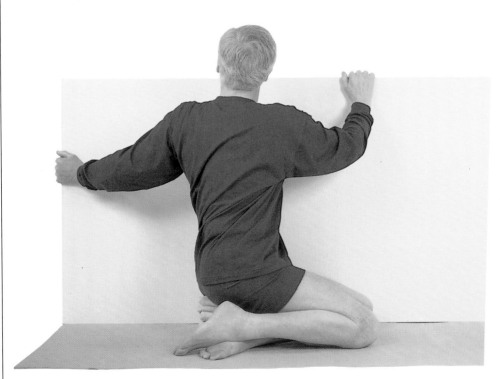

2 *Turn toward the ledge, gripping it with both hands to help you turn as far as you can.* | *Turn the shoulders and chest. Stay for 20–30 seconds, then repeat on the other side.*

MARICYASANA III
—TWIST WITH OPPOSITE ARM AGAINST LEG—

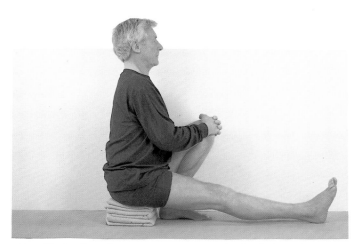 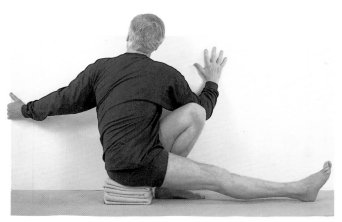

1 Sit in Dandasana (no. 18) with the left side against a wall or ledge. Bend the left leg up and bring the foot close to its own thigh. Hold the knee and stretch the trunk up.

2 Turn the trunk toward the wall. Bring the right elbow to the outer edge of the left knee, fix the upper arm firmly against the knee and hold the ledge. Use the hands to help you turn as far as you can. Stay for 20–30 seconds, then repeat on the other side.

SETU BANDHA SARVANGASANA
—NECK BALANCE BACK ARCH—

Do Setu Bandha Sarvangasana (no. 39), variant on bench.

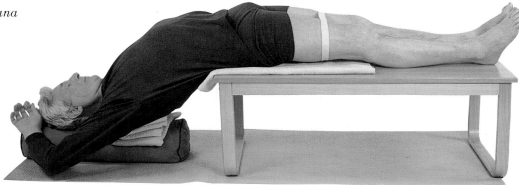

SAVASANA
—CORPSE POSE—

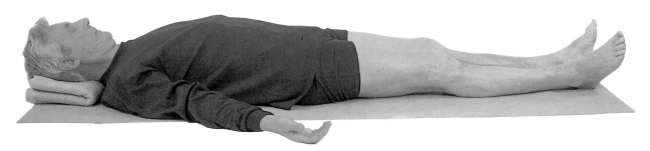

Do Savasana (no. 41). Stay for 5–10 minutes, then turn to the side and get up.

ASANAS FOR BACKACHE

The postures given in this programme are designed to alleviate simple backaches, both of the lower and the upper back. They are not, however, intended for severe conditions such as slipped disc or pain resulting from a fracture or other medical problem; in these cases advice should be sought from a teacher experienced in yoga therapy.

The postures are all suitable for beginners. With continued practice, back problems should decrease and may disappear altogether. The back should become stronger and less liable to ache.

When doing the postures, do not jerk or move suddenly. Keep the affected part passive and move below or above it. Do not focus on the painful part directly. In the beginning, the painful part needs to be rested, not worked.

HALF UTTANASANA
— HALF FORWARD BEND —

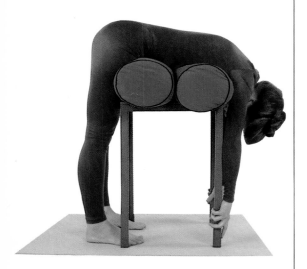

Stand in front of a tall stool or small table. Place neatly folded blankets or bolsters on it to raise the height to that of your hips. Take the feet about hip-width apart. Stand on tip-toe and bend over the stool, tucking the edge of the blankets or bolster into the groin. Extend the abdomen and the front ribs over the bolster. Then stretch the heels to touch the ground. Relax the arms down, or hold the legs of the stool. Keep the legs vertical. Allow the spine and back ribs to relax.

Stay for 30–60 seconds. Come up carefully.

BHARADVAJASANA ON CHAIR
CHAIR TWIST

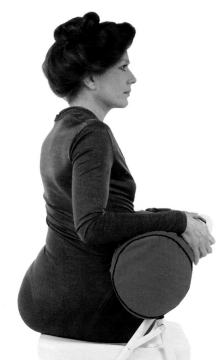

Sit sideways on a chair. Stretch the trunk up. Take one or two breaths. Turn toward the back of the chair. Place a bolster or folded blankets between the back of the chair and the abdomen. Grip the back of the chair and turn as far as possible. Do not hold the breath.

Stay for 20–30 seconds, then repeat on the other side.

FORWARD BEND

Sit on the chair and spread the legs apart. Place a bolster or folded blanket across the thighs, tucking it into the groin. Extend the abdomen and the front ribs over it. Bend down. Take the arms inside the legs of the chair and hold the back legs of the chair. Relax the head.

Stay for 20–30 seconds. Come up carefully, without jerking.

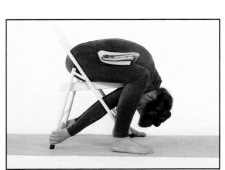

MARICYASANA (STANDING)
— STANDING TWIST —

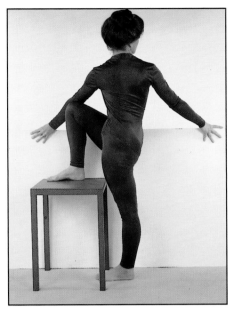

Do Maricyasana (standing) (no. 32). Stay for 20–30 seconds, then repeat on the other side.

PARSVA PAVANA MUKTASANA
— WIND RELEASING POSE —

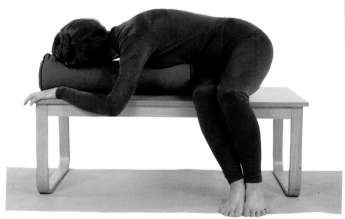

Sit at the left side of a low bench or sturdy coffee table. Place a bolster or folded blankets lengthwise on top of it, to your right. Turn toward the bolster. Bend down and rest the length of the front of the body along it. Hold the bench or bolster and turn the head to the right. Keep the legs facing forward as much as possible. Extend the front ribs and relax the back.

Stay for 30–60 seconds, then repeat on the other side. After bending to the sides, do Pavana Muktasana: sit at the front of the bench, spread the knees apart and bend down. If bending is easy, it is a sign of recovery.

UTTHITA TRIKONASANA
— EXTENDED TRIANGLE POSE —

Do Trikonasana (no. 3) with the back against a wall. If possible, find a wall with a projecting corner so that you can hold it.

Stay for 20–30 seconds, then repeat on the other side.

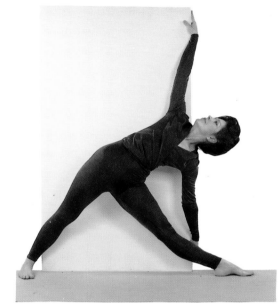

ARDHA CANDRASANA
— HALF-MOON POSE —

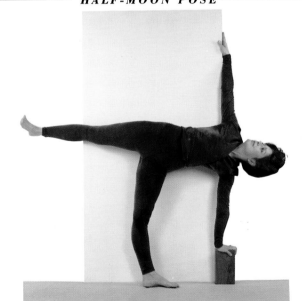

Do Ardha Candrasana against the wall (see "Asanas for Stiff Hips"). Hold on to a projecting corner of a wall with the top hand. Place the lower hand on a block and the raised heel on the wall. Turn the trunk upward.

Stay for 20–30 seconds, then repeat on the other side.

● *If you have sciatica, turn the front foot out 120°.*

PARSVOTTANASANA
— SIDEWAYS STRETCH —

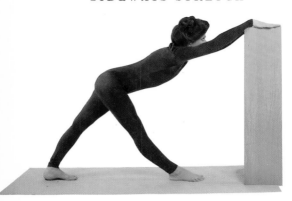

Do Parsvottanasana (no. 7) as follows: stand in Tadasana (no. 1) about 3 ft (90 cm) from a ledge with your right side facing it. Take the feet 3¹⁄₂–4 ft (105–120 cm) apart. Turn the left foot 45°–60° in and the right foot 90° out. Turn the trunk to face the ledge. Bring the left hip forward in line with the right. Bend down and place the hands on the ledge. Straighten the arms. Keep the hips level and the legs straight. Stretch the trunk.

Stay for 20–30 seconds, then repeat on the other side.

UTTANASANA
FORWARD EXTENSION
— ON LEDGE —

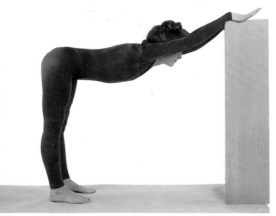

Do Uttanasana (variant on ledge) (no. 9). Stay for 20–30 seconds, then come up.

ADHO MUKHA SVANASANA
— DOG POSE HEAD DOWN —

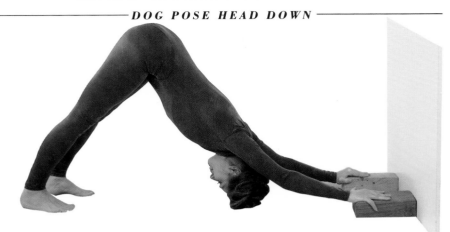

Do Adho Mukha Svanasana (no. 31) as follows: place two blocks against a wall about 18 inches (45 cm) or shoulder-width apart. Kneel down and place the hands on the blocks. Raise the hips and straighten the arms and legs to make an inverted "V" shape. If necessary, walk the feet further back. Keep the hips up. Stretch the arms and trunk up, away from the blocks. Relax the head.

Stay for 20–30 seconds, then come down.

VIRASANA FORWARD BEND
— HERO POSE —

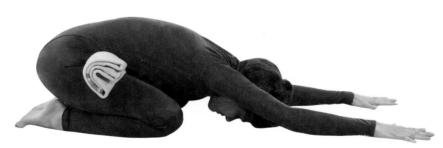

Do Virasana Forward Bend (no. 16) as follows: place a rolled or folded blanket on the thighs and tuck it into the groin. Extend the abdomen over it.

Stay for 30–60 seconds.

SUKHASANA (WITH SIDEWAYS BEND)
— EASY POSE —

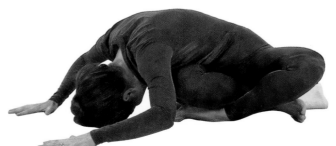

Sit in Sukhasana (no. 14) with the legs crossed simply. Turn to the right and bend down over the right leg. Stay for 30–60 seconds, then change the cross legs and bend to the right.

ARDHA HALASANA
— *HALF-PLOUGH POSE* —

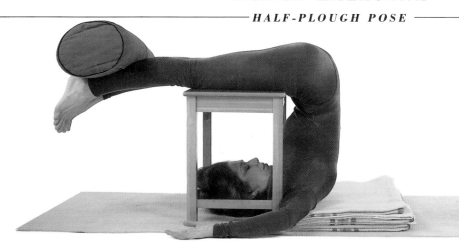

Do Ardha Halasana (no. 36). If possible, ask someone to place a weight such as a bolster or pile of blankets on the lower calves.

Stay for 5–8 minutes, then remove the bolster and slide down.

SUPTA PADANGUSTHASANA
— *RECLINING FINGER-TO-FOOT POSE* —

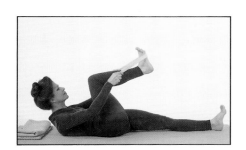

1 *Lie on the floor in a straight line. If necessary, place a blanket under the head. Bend the right leg over the abdomen and place a belt round the foot.*

2 *Hold the belt with both hands and straighten the right leg up. Press the left thigh down. Stretch the left leg along the floor and the right leg up.*

Stay for 20–30 seconds, then bend the right leg and bring it down. Line yourself up again and repeat on the other side.

VARIANT

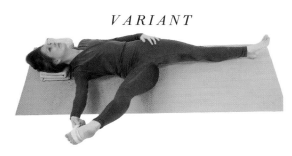

Lie in a straight line. Follow the method given in steps 1 and 2.

Press the left thigh down with the left hand. Raise and straighten the right leg, then turn it outward and take it down to the right. Keep both legs stretched.

Stay for 20–30 seconds. Raise the leg, bend it and lower it to the floor. Repeat on the other side.

SAVASANA
— *CORPSE POSE* —

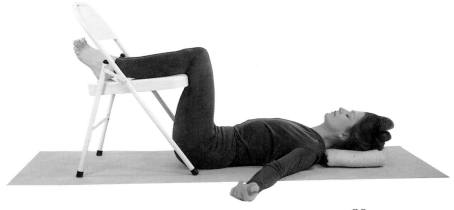

Do Savasana (no. 41) as follows: bend the legs and rest the calves on a stool or chair. Relax.

Stay for 5–10 minutes. Bring the legs down, turn to the side and get up carefully.

ASANAS FOR STIFF HIPS

The sequence of postures in this programme is designed to make the hips and lower back work more efficiently, by increasing mobility and strength. Too often the hip and sacro-iliac joints become stiff through incorrect use, or under- or over use. Often they become affected by arthritic conditions. Ease of movement of these joints is important, especially in later life when ordinary movements, such as sitting, standing and walking, may become slow and difficult. Yoga postures are an invaluable tool to prevent this.

BHARADVAJASANA (ON CHAIR)
CHAIR TWIST

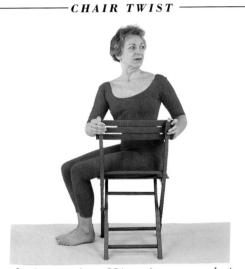

Do Bharadvajasana (no. 33) variant on a chair. Stay for 20–30 seconds, then repeat on the other side.

UTTHITA TRIKONASANA
TRIANGLE POSE

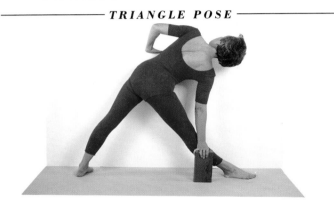

Do Trikonasana (no. 3), facing a wall or ledge. Place a block by the outer edge of the right foot and put your hand on it. Grip the wall or ledge with the left hand. Use the hands to help you to turn the trunk toward the wall and press the right hip forward. Stay for 20–30 seconds, then repeat on the other side.

MARICYASANA (STANDING)

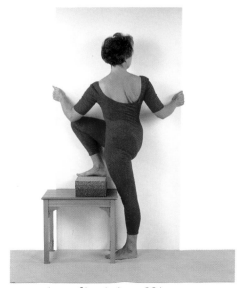

Do Maricyasana (standing) (no. 32).

UTTHITA PARSVAKONASANA
LATERAL ANGLE POSE

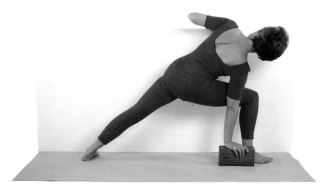

Do Parsvakonasana (no. 4) facing a wall or ledge. Place a block on the floor by the right foot and place your hand on it. With the left hand, grip the ledge or press the wall. Lift the right hip and press it toward the wall. Turn the trunk toward the wall, with the hands. Stay for 20–30 seconds, then repeat on the other side.

VIRABHADRASANA I
——— WARRIOR POSE I ———

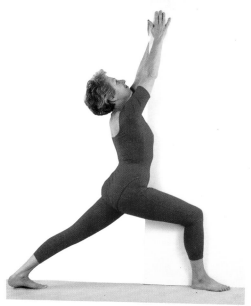

PARIVRTTA TRIKONASANA
REVERSE TRIANGLE POSE

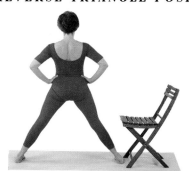

1 Stand in Tadasana (no. 1) with a chair placed about 3 ft (105 cm) to your right. Place the hands on the hips and spread the legs 3¹/₂–4 ft (90–120 cm) apart.

Do Virabhadrasana I (no. 5) as follows: stand sideways in a doorway facing the door post (or face a column). Hold it and take the right leg forward along the wall, with the inner thigh touching the door post. Bend the knee to a right angle. Step back with the left leg and straighten it. If necessary, raise the heel. Turn the hips and pelvis toward the post and stretch the front of the body up against it. Press the lower back (sacrum) toward the post, without raising the right hip. Take the hands higher to gain the maximum stretch. Stay for 20–30 seconds, then repeat on the other side.

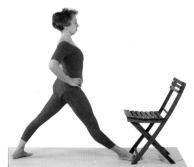

2 Turn the left foot 45–60° in and the right foot 90° out. Turn the hips and trunk to the right.

VIRABHADRASANA II
——— WARRIOR POSE II ———

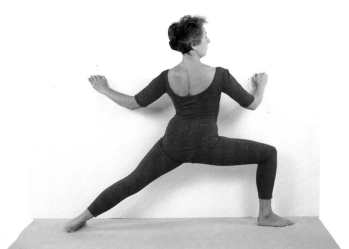

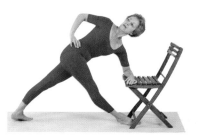

3 Revolve the trunk further and take it down toward the chair, so that the left side faces the floor and the right side faces the ceiling. Rest the left forearm on the seat of the chair and grip the edge. Keep the right hand on the hip. Extend the trunk and turn the hips and trunk as far as you can. Stay for 20–30 seconds, then repeat on the other side.

Do Virabhadrasana II (no. 6) facing a wall or a ledge. Hold the ledge firmly. Press the right hip toward the wall and move the right knee away from it. Stay for 20–30 seconds. Repeat on the other side.

UTTHITA HASTA PADANGUSTHASANA

EXTENDED LEG RAISING

All three variants should be practised.

FORWARD	*SIDEWAYS*	*TWIST*

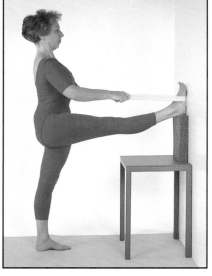 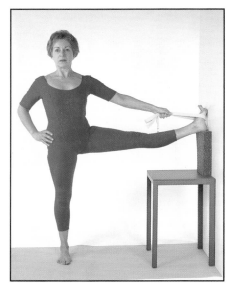 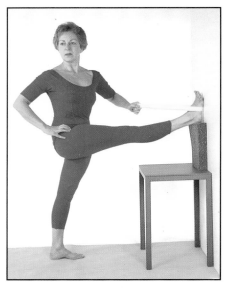

Place a high stool against a wall. Do Utthita Hasta Padangusthasana (no. 13) forward, using a belt to hold the raised foot. Stretch the trunk up. Stay for 30–60 seconds, then repeat on the other side.	*Place a high stool against a wall. Do Utthita Hasta Padangusthasana (no. 13) sideways, using a belt to hold the raised foot. Stretch the trunk up. Stay for 30–60 seconds, then repeat on the other side.*	*Stand in Tadasana (no. 1), facing the wall. Raise the right foot on to a stool. Straighten both the legs. Hold the belt with the left hand, place the right hand on the right hip and turn the trunk to the right. Stay for 20–30 seconds, then repeat on the other side.*

SARVANGASANA (ON WALL)

NECK BALANCE ON WALL

Do Sarvangasana against a wall (no. 38). Stay for 3–5 minutes, then bend the legs and come down.

BHARADVAJASANA

SIMPLE TWIST

Do Bharadvajasana (no. 33) with the hands against a wall to help you twist. Stay for 20–30 seconds, then repeat on the other side.

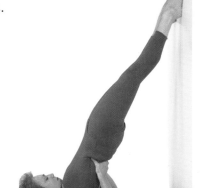

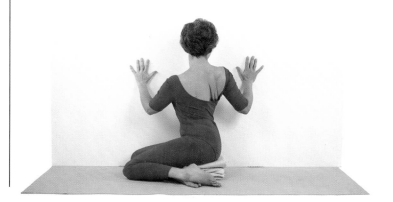

SUPTA PADANGUSTHASANA
──────── RECLINING FINGER-TO-FOOT POSE ────────

All three variants should be practised.

LEG UP

Lie near a column or door post. Bend the left leg and take it up against the post, at 90° to the ground. Support the whole leg, from the buttock to the heel. Extend the right leg along the floor. Stay for 30–60 seconds, then repeat on the other side.

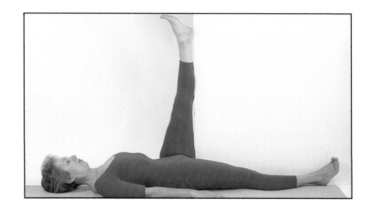

LEG SIDEWAYS

Lie on the floor with the feet against a wall. Bend the left leg over the abdomen and place a belt around the foot. Raise and straighten the leg, then turn it outward in its socket and take it down to the left. Rest the foot on a block or pile of books. Stay for 30–60 seconds, then repeat on the other side.

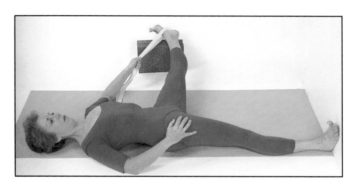

LEG ACROSS

Lie on the floor with the feet against a wall. Bend the right leg, put a belt round the foot and hold it. Straighten the leg, then hold the belt with the left hand and take the leg sideways down to the left. Do not let the left leg turn inward. Stay for 30–60 seconds, then repeat on the other side.

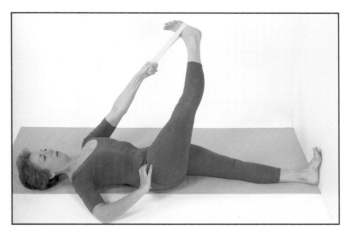

SAVASANA
──────── CORPSE POSE ────────

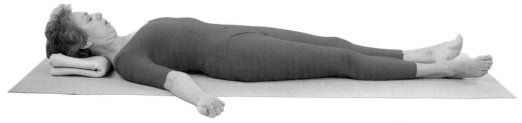

Do Savasana (no. 41). Stay for 5–10 minutes, then turn to the side and get up.

NAMES OF THE POSTURES

Yoga postures are all named in Sanskrit, the classical language of India. In the Asanas section, an English equivalent has been given, either in a direct translation or a description.

The names have been transliterated according to international convention, but omitting the relevant diacritical marks. However, to help readers who wish to learn the correct pronunciation, the postures and other Sanskrit words that appear in the text are listed here with their diacritical marks.

The following points should be noted:

Stress: This is usually on the first syllable. The ā of āsana is always stressed.

Vowels: Long vowels are indicated by a bar over the letter.

Consonants:
c is pronounced "ch".
ś and ṣ are pronounced "sh".
h following any consonant (kh, gh, ph, bh, ch) should be pronounced

distinctly to differentiate it from unaspirated consonants.

ṭ, ḍ, ṇ, are pronounced retroflexively (with the tongue curled back).

ṛ is a semivowel, pronounced as a combination of r and i.

ṅ precedes k or g.

ñ precedes c or j.

A more complete guide to pronunciation can be found in *Light on Yoga* and *Yoga: The Iyengar Way* (see Further Reading).

Adho Mukha Śvānāsana
Ardha Baddha Padma
  Paścimottānāsana
Ardha Candrāsana
Ardha Halāsana
Baddhakonāsana
Bhāradvājāsana
Daṇḍāsana
Garuḍāsata
Gomukhāsana
Halāsana
Jānuśīrṣāsana

Mālāsana
Marīcyāsana
Matsyāsana
Pādāṅguṣṭhāsana
Parsva Pavana
  Muktāsana
Pārśvottānāsana
Parvatāsana
Paścimottānāsana
Prāsarita Pādottānāsana
Sarvāṅgāsana
Śavāsana

Setu Bandha Sarvāṅgāsana
Siddhāsana
Sukhāsana
Supta Baddhakonāsana
Supta Pādāṅguṣṭhāsana
Supta Vīrāsana
Tāḍāsana
Triaṅ Mukhaikapāda
  Paścimottānāsana
Upavistakonāsana
Ūrdhva Prasārita Pādāsana
Utkaṭāsana

Uttānāsana
Utthita Hasta
  Pādāṅguṣṭhāsana
Utthita Pārśvakoṇāsana
Utthita Trikoṇāsana
Viparīta Karaṇī
Vīrabhadrāsana I
Vīrabhadrāsana II
Vīrāsana
Vṛkṣasana

FURTHER READING

B. K. S. Iyengar, *Light on Yoga*. Allen and Unwin, 1966

Light on Pranayama, Allen and Unwin, 1981

The Illustrated Light on Yoga (formerly *The Concise Light on Yoga*, Allen and Unwin, 1980), Harper Collins, 1993

Light on the Yoga Sutras of Patanjali, Harper Collins, 1993

The Tree of Yoga, Fine Line Books, 1988

Geeta S. Iyengar, *Yoga: A Gem for Women*, Allied Publishers, 1983

Silva, Mira and Shyam Mehta, *Yoga: The Iyengar Way*, Dorling Kindersley, 1990

The Upanisads (any edition)

The Bhagavad Gita (any edition)

USEFUL ADDRESSES

Contact the centres listed for information about local Institutes.

UK

Iyengar Yoga Institute
223A Randolph Avenue
London W9 1NL

Manchester & District Institute of Iyengar Yoga
134 King Street
Dukinfield
Tameside
Greater Manchester

Edinburgh Iyengar Yoga Centre
195 Bruntsfield Place
Edinburgh EH10 4DQ

US

BKS Iyengar Yoga National Association of the United States, Incorporated
8223 W. Third Street
Los Angeles
CA 90038

Iyengar Yoga Association of Northern California
2404 27th Avenue
San Francisco
CA 94116

Iyengar Yoga Institute of New York
27 W. 24th Street
Suite 800
New York
NY 10011

Iyengar Yoga Association of Massachusetts, Inc.
240-A Elm Street
Somerville
MA 02114

Iyengar Yoga Association of Minnesota
Box 10381
Minneapolis
MN 55458-3381

Iyengar Yoga Association of Wisconsin
Route 2
Box 70E
La Crosse
WI 54601

Iyengar Yoga Association of the Midwest Bioregions
310 Gralake
Ann Arbor
MI 48103

CANADA

BKS Iyengar Yoga Association
27-F Meadowlark Village
Edmonton
Alberta
T5R 5X4

Centre de Yoga Iyengar de Montreal
919 Mont-Royal Oest
Montreal
PQ H2J 1X3

BKS Iyengar Yoga Association
PO 65694, Station F
Vancouver, BC
V4N 5K7

BKS Iyengar Yoga Association of Ontario
c/o 85 Glenforest Road
Toronto
Ontario
M4N 2A1

AUSTRALIA

BKS Iyengar Association of Australasia
1 Rickman Avenue
Mosman 2088
N.S.W.

Bondi Junction School of Yoga
First Floor
2A Waverly Street
Bondi Junction
Sydney 202
N.S.W.

INDIA

R.I.M. Yoga Institute
1107 B/1 Shivajinagar
Pune 411 016

SOUTH AFRICA

BKS Iyengar Institute
58 Trelawney Road
Pietermaritzburg
Natal 3201

Iyengar Yoga Association of S. Africa
PO Box 78648
Sandton 2146

INDEX